DATE DUE

MY 18 '05		
OCT 18 2008	NOV 06 2017	
OCT 22 2008		
OCT 5 2009		
FE 16 '10		
FE 25 '10		
OCT 06 2010		
MAR 02 2011		
FEB 20 2013		
OCT 23 2013		
MAR 17 2014		
MAY 26 2017		
OCT 04 2017		

Hallucinogens

A Reader

Charles S. Grob, M.D.

Jeremy P. Tarcher / Putnam
a member of Penguin Putnam Inc.
New York

Most Tarcher/Putnam books are available at special quantity discounts for bulk purchase for sales promotions, premiums, fund-raising, and educational needs. Special books or book excerpts also can be created to fit specific needs. For details, write Putnam Special Markets, 375 Hudson Street, New York, NY 10014.

Jeremy P. Tarcher/Putnam
a member of
Penguin Putnam Inc.
375 Hudson Street
New York, NY 10014
www.penguinputnam.com

Library of Congress Cataloging-in-Publication Data

Hallucinogens : a reader / [compiled by] Charles S. Grob.
p.   cm.
ISBN 1-58542-166-9
1. Hallucinogenic drugs.   I. Grob, Charles S., date.
RM324.8 H345   2002   2001057402
615'.7883—dc21

Printed in the United States of America

1   3   5   7   9   10   8   6   4   2

Book design by Lovedog Studio

This book is dedicated to my mother,
Elizabeth Grob (1924–1998),
who taught me to tell it like it is,
and to my father, David Grob (1919–   ),
who told me to write what I had to say.

Acknowledgments

OVER THE YEARS I have had the good fortune to be associated with a great many people who have supported my endeavors and my goals. I would like to express my gratitude to those whom I have met and interacted with on the path. Neither this book nor whatever else I have contributed would ever have occurred without their support. In particular, I want to thank Jeremy Tarcher for his patience in allowing this project to unfold, some years beyond its projected submission date, and for his referral to me of Mark Waldman, without whose expert editorial guidance and help in getting organized this book could not have been completed.

I also want to acknowledge the many friends and colleagues who have shared an appreciation and vision that the hallucinogens possess untapped potential for modern science and culture, including fellow board members of the Heffter Research Institute, David Nichols, Mark Geyer, George Greer, Dennis McKenna, Jerry Patchen, Franz Vollenweider and Bob Wallace, as well as James Thornton and Lynette Herring; Rick Doblin and Sylvia Thyssen of MAPS; Robert Jesse of the Council on Spiritual Practices, and Jace Callaway, Glacus de Souza Brito, Marlene De Rios, Alexander Shulgin, Frances Vaughan, David Presti, Joel Alter, Jarvin Heiman, Phil Baum, Malcolm Groome, Sidney Sudberg, Betsy Gordon and Alise Agar.

I would also like to extend my deep appreciation to the late Alexander Rogawaski of Los Angeles and to Joseph Coyle, formerly of The Johns Hopkins Hospital in Baltimore, for their valued mentorship during my training in psychiatry and child psychiatry, and to Milton Miller and Ira Lesser for creating a work environment at Harbor-UCLA Medical Center that fosters commitment and productivity.

I am grateful to Gary Bravo and Susan Seitz for their close friendship and their aid in helping me keep my sense of humor and proportion during life's trials and tribulations. Finally, my acknowledgments would not be complete without expressing gratitude to Anne and Stephanie for their love, tolerance and editorial insight.

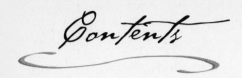

Contents

Appendix C

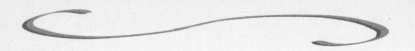

All the vegetable sedatives and narcotics, all the euphorics that grow on trees, the hallucinogens that ripen in berries or can be squeezed from roots—all, without exception, have been known and systematically used by human beings from time immemorial.

—ALDOUS HUXLEY, 1954

Psychedelic experience is only a glimpse of genuine mystical insight, but a glimpse which can be matured and deepened by the various ways of meditation in which drugs are no longer necessary or useful. When you get the message, hang up the phone. For psychedelic drugs are simply instruments, like microscopes, telescopes, and telephones. The biologist does not sit with eye permanently glued to the microscope; he goes away and works on what he has seen.

—ALAN WATTS, 1962

The forlornness of consciousness in our world is due primarily to the loss of instinct, and the reason for this lies in the development of the human mind over the past aeon. The more power man had over nature, the more his knowledge and skill went to his head, and the deeper became his contempt for the merely natural.

—CARL JUNG, 1957

If the doors of perception were cleansed every
thing would appear to man as it is, infinite.
For man has closed himself up, till he sees all
things thro' narrow chinks of his cavern.

—WILLIAM BLAKE, 1793

This we know: All things are connected
Like the blood which unites one family.
All things are connected.
Whatever befalls the earth
Befalls the sons of the earth.
Man did not weave the web of life.
He is merely a strand in it.
Whatever he does to the web
He does to himself.

—CHIEF SEATTLE, 1856

Hallucinogens Revisited

Charles S. Grob, M.D.

IT HAS BEEN forty years since Timothy Leary heard about the magic mushrooms of Northern Mexico from his friend and colleague Frank Barron. That fateful day, in the summer of 1960, by a swimming pool in the Mexican city of Cuernavaca, Leary ingested several grams of the genus *Stropharia cubensis* and experienced a dazzling and unprecedented perceptual display of visions that resulted in a profound reorganization of his core sense of self. Unaware of the long and (by necessity) often secret history of hallucinogens in both the New and Old Worlds, Leary returned to his teaching post at the Harvard University Department of Social Relations intent upon developing an entirely novel research program studying the effects of these compounds on the human psyche. What followed is the regrettable saga of a brilliant academic, having discovered a potentially valuable tool for remodeling personality, running headlong into a culture ill-prepared for radical change and increasingly antagonistic to his provocative herald of the *New Age*.

What Leary failed to appreciate, amid the excitement of presenting his breakthrough discoveries initially to his Harvard colleagues and students and later through the media to the world, was the ingrained resistance he would encounter. These extraordinary plants and synthetic substances, which so delighted his senses and fascinated his intellect, would be repelled by a mainstream culture that saw in them the manifestation of a perfidious threat to social stability. Leary himself became the embodiment of these fears, and spurred on by his own recklessness and confrontational nature, was repudiated, attacked and ultimately victimized by the champions of the status quo. To no small degree, the monolithic *War On Drugs* was a direct consequence of the perceived threat Timothy Leary and his associates posed during the brief ascendancy of the 1960s counter-culture. In January, 1968, President Lyndon Johnson, in his State of the Union address, warned against "these powders and pills which threaten our nation's health, vitality and self-respect." Later condemned as "Public Enemy Number One" by Johnson's successor, Richard Nixon, Leary was forcibly removed from the forum of public ideas and civic discourse. In the wake of his subsequent imprisonment, self-imposed exile and eventual cultural marginalization, Leary's passage through time paralleled the fate of those psychoactive substances he was so closely identified with.

The world we live in today is not the same as the one in which Leary so strongly excited passions. The divisive atmosphere which once pitted the leaders of the counterculture against the defenders of the faith has receded. Such issues as minority rights and gender equality, once standards of the politically radical fringe, have now generally been accepted into the mainstream of politics and education. The question of the hallucinogens, however, remains split off and feared, rarely discussed in the forum of public ideas. Though recognized by some as catalyzing much of the progressive shifts our culture has undergone since the 1960s, the hallucinogens themselves have received scant attention. In a society purporting openness and receptivity to new ideas and innovative tools, this persistent denial and avoidance of serious dialogue is troubling.

The question before us now is: Are we, as a culture, ready to seriously reevaluate the intrinsic properties and potentials of this often misunderstood class of drugs? The time has come to put Timothy Leary and his much maligned legacy to rest, and to open the doors once again to a fair and objective inquiry into the potential risks *and* benefits of hallucinogens. It has been forty years since Leary's encounter with the *magic mushrooms* of Mexico. But have we matured enough as a culture to reopen this dialogue and debate? If so, then we have before us a fascinating and potentially valuable and enriching path. However, if we have not achieved the moral and psychological level of stability essential for this work, then this remarkable opportunity will once again be lost.

An alternative model to Leary's notorious *turn on, tune in and drop out* was proposed by the brilliant British writer and intellectual Aldous Huxley. Long intrigued by psychoactive compounds and their capacity to mold human personality, Huxley in his classic 1932 novel *Brave New World* depicted a society centered around the dehumanizing and conditioning effects of the fictional drug *Soma*. Throughout his career, Huxley maintained his interest in the developing field of psychopharmacology. In his classic 1957 article *Brave New World Revisited*, published in the *Saturday Evening Post*, he described his fascination with the capacity of drugs to influence personality, for better or for worse. While living in Los Angeles in 1954, Huxley was introduced to mescaline, the potent active alkaloid of the peyote plant. Guided by the Canadian psychiatric researcher Humphry Osmond, Huxley's extraordinary inner voyage led him to believe that he had witnessed the necessary next step for human evolution. Expanding upon his ideas and revelations in *Doors of Perception* and *Heaven and Hell*, his writings awakened interest in this hitherto little-known phenomenon.

Huxley perceived the threshold of a new era in which the effects of these extraordinary substances would catalyze an age of creative expression and world peace. The Huxley paradigm for the optimal integration of hallucinogens into society called for their discrete introduction to the cultural leaders of the day, in contrast to Leary's promotion of mass consumption by the general public. With this in mind, Huxley visited Leary at Harvard to attempt to convince him to work quietly with these powerful substances. Inevitably, Huxley's mission failed. Even so, it is unlikely that history's fate for the hallucinogens could have been altered, given the rapid spread of knowledge of their existence. From Boston to Los Angeles, and across the oceans, word was out. No doubt, if Timothy Leary had never existed, the culture would have had to invent some other challenging visionary to assume the role of bringing hallucinogens to public consciousness, and paying the price for it.

In 1962 Huxley published his final book, *Island*. In it, he wrote passionately about the myriad possibilities he beheld within the realm of the hallucinogens. The novel tells the tale of the mythic island of Pala, where social cohesion and moral knowledge are conveyed and internalized through the ritual use of a fictional plant hallucinogen, *Moksha* (Sanskrit for "liberation"). The story proposes the ideal context within which these sacred substances could be incorporated into society. However, Huxley understood that modern society was not ready to embrace this vision. He ended his story tragically, as the island, Pala, is invaded and overwhelmed by its rapacious and warlike neighbor, the powerful country of Rendang. The story serves as a metaphor dramatizing Huxley's belief that the contemporary mainstream culture of his time was not prepared for the introduction of these long-secret tools of the ancient world. Aversion and repudiation would be the fate of the hallucinogens, and their innate capacity to heal and to inform would remain untapped for years.

On November 22, 1963, the day of President John Kennedy's assassination, Huxley died of metastatic cancer. He had remained until the end consistent in his faith in hallucinogens, and in their ability to assist an individual's passage from life into death. As he approached the moment of death, on prearranged signal with his wife, Laura, and his personal physician, Huxley was administered an injection of 100 micrograms of lysergic acid diethylamide (LSD).

Reopening the Doors of Perception

It may be possible once again to revisit the legendary *Moksha* Medicine of Huxley's *Island,* this time within the context of a contemporary world that respects their careful and objective exploration. If this is to be done, it is imperative that attention be given to the lessons of the past. What can be learned from the unfortunate saga of Timothy Leary and his age, or for that matter of the tragic fate of Huxley's *Island?* To understand what went wrong, it is necessary to comprehend the ancient roots of the hallucinogens. Mounting evidence within the fields of anthropology, comparative religion and ethnobotany point to widespread prehistorical existence of tribal communities where shamanic practices incorporated socially sanctioned rituals with plant hallucinogens. These rituals not only became the bedrock upon which beliefs and identities were forged, but also contained important rules of conduct which ensured the safety of all individuals within the community. Hallucinogens were perceived of as being sacred, put on the earth by the Supreme Being(s) to allow communion between the spirit and the material worlds for the purposes of healing and divination. These substances were not taken for recreational or frivolous purposes, nor were they taken outside of strict ritual context. In contrast, contemporary use of hallucinogens often distorts ancient traditions, compromises inherent safeguards and sets the stage for dangerous abuse. The challenge for today is to determine if and how these substances would have a healing role in our society. By adapting ancient practices to conform to our own contemporary setting, might we glean the benefits once enjoyed by ancient communities?

Science, and particularly the fields of medicine and psychiatry, has too long neglected these drugs. Frightened by the cultural reactions and upheaval of the 1960s, once-thriving research programs were forced to terminate their activities. The involvement of biased political agendas with scientific policy has further obstructed progress. Though once on the cutting edge of psychiatric research, the historical role of hallucinogens has been increasingly denied. Since the early 1980s, references to these substances have been virtually excluded from the curriculum of residency training programs. Many psychiatrists today are completely unaware of this history. This is unfortunate, as what has been forgotten is the potential for hallucinogens to facilitate healing, particularly in psychiatric patients nonresponsive to conventional treatment modalities. If modern psychiatry continues to ignore the challenges of exploring the range of effects these substances induce, the field and the people it serves will ultimately be done a great disservice.

In the future, a wide range of applications and research paradigms await. Utilizing today's state-of-the-art technologies, fascinating new knowledge on how the brain functions will be acquired. Tremendous potentials also lie before us in the development of innovative treatment programs. While conventional psychopharmacology relies upon the daily administration of expensive medication, often for months or years, the hallucinogen facilitated treatment model offers an alternative. It calls for only one or perhaps a handful of augmented treatment sessions stretched out over time within the context of ongoing psychotherapy. Various conditions, including the pain and distress of dying, substance abuse disorders, chronic post-traumatic stress disorder and numerous others, often resistant to current treatment, may prove to be amenable to this novel paradigm for healing.

Preliminary results from the golden era of hallucinogen research in the 1950s and 1960s offer substantial reason for optimism. Early findings established that once supported by formal research, hallucinogen facilitated interventions often demonstrated positive ranges of safety and therapeutic efficacy. There has been a long hiatus in the study of these unusual psychoactive compounds. We now have the opportunity to develop investigations utilizing the current research methodologies and technologies of the twenty-first century. Inevitably, the barriers to conducting carefully designed approved research examining the hallucinogen treatment model will be removed, at which time the fields of psychiatry and medicine may begin to evolve in new and intriguing directions.

New Research

Over the last decade, progress has been made establishing the foundation for a new generation of sanctioned research studies with hallucinogens. A variety of compounds, including dimethyltryptamine (DMT), 3,4-methylenedioxymethamphetamine (MDMA) and ibogaine have been subjected to rigorous Phase 1 testing in normal volunteers. In Europe, particularly in Switzerland, considerable progress has occurred in establishing a foundation of basic physiological and psychological responses to hallucinogen administration. And in South America, field research of Amazonian plant hallucinogens has yielded new information.

Although government research funding agencies have been reluctant to offer much support, small private foundations have succeeded in generating the momentum necessary for progress to occur. In the United States, the Heffter Research Institute and the Multidisciplinary Association for Psychedelic Studies (MAPS) are dedicated to establishing methods of investigation which adhere to the highest standards of academic research. These two organizations have developed core groups of neuroscientists and psychiatrists who provide critical advice and guidance to investigators seeking funding and regulatory approvals.

In the early 1990s, I was granted federal, state and institutional approval to study the effects of MDMA (3,4-methylenedioxymethamphetamine) upon a group of healthy volunteers, examining changes in body temperature, blood pressure, heart rate, the neuroendocrine system and observable psychological effects. In addition, brain function was studied using state-of-the-art imaging technologies. During our investigations on the Clinical Research Unit at Harbor-UCLA Medical Center, our volunteers were given, on three separate occasions, an experimental dose of either MDMA or a placebo. All subjects reported having a positive psychological response, except one. This individual, who was participating in his first experimental session, became moderately agitated and complained of high levels of anxiety and emotional distress that he attributed to the hospital setting. He stated that he was extremely sensitive, "picking up on all the negative vibes of the hospital." The subject was asked to abide by the rules he had consented to. He was required to remain in the hospital through the night, but he could drop out of the study and leave the following morning. The subject eagerly agreed to that option, and withdrew from the program the next day. After the subject left the study, we discovered, to our great surprise, that he had actually been given an inactive placebo. This was the only negative psychological experience reported during our study, and it taught a good lesson about the power of the placebo response.

One other young man experienced an adverse medical reaction. He had already participated in the first two experimental sessions, without difficulty, but on his third and final occasion, he experienced, within an hour after taking the experimental drug, a dramatic elevation of blood pressure. Upon questioning about what could have been "different" that morning compared to the other two occasions, the young man stated that he had spent the night before at the house of a friend who lived close to the hospital. The friend apparently had a cat, to which the subject reportedly had an allergic reaction. To remedy this problem, he took some of his friend's asthma medicine, which in combination with the experimental medicine, caused a significant elevation in blood pressure. Although the man's blood pressure gradually subsided and returned to baseline after about an hour, and he sustained no apparent lingering medical complication from the event, this episode does highlight the concern that some recreational users of "Ecstasy" (which often, though not always, contains MDMA), who also may be taking prescription medications or illicit drugs, could induce potentially dangerous drug interactions. There was a lot to be learned from these two subjects, as the nature of their experiences both highlights critical parameters for future clinical treatment investigations and directs our attention to the important public health questions surrounding the recreational use of MDMA.

Another opportunity to engage in collaborative research with hallucinogens presented itself in 1993. I was invited to Manaus, in the Brazilian Amazon, to join a team of scientists from the departments of medicine and psychiatry at the Universidade do Amazonas, the Universidade Estadual do Rio de Janeiro, and the Escola Paulista de Medicina do Sao Paulo. We conducted a series of Phase 1 investigations on a randomly recruited group of 15 male subjects. These men, all members of the syncretic church Uniao do Vegetal, had consumed ayahuasca (a powerful plant hallucinogen) for at least the past ten years as part of religious ritual ceremonies. For comparative reasons, our study also evaluated fifteen matched control subjects who had never taken ayahuasca. Our findings, which were published in respected professional journals, including *Psychopharmacology* (116:385–387, 1994), the *Journal of Nervous and Mental Disease* (184:86–94, 1996) and the *Journal of Ethnopharmacology* (65:243–256, 1999), demonstrated higher levels of psychological and physical health in ayahuasca subjects as compared to control subjects who had never experienced ayahuasca. We also found that the subjects who attended ayahuasca ceremonies had unusually large numbers of serotonin receptors (a neurotransmitter involved in the regulation of mood). This led us to believe that this particular plant hallucinogen concoction may be more effective in treating and preventing certain types of depression and other psychiatric conditions than our current paradigm of using prescription drugs. In the future, we hope to continue our studies with this mysterious South American plant medicine.

During my visit to Manaus, I acquired an appreciation of the life-transforming experiences these subjects had undergone. Many of the men, before joining the ayahuasca church, had severe drug and alcohol disorders, but since their involvement had maintained absolute sobriety for all substances other than ayahuasca, which was used under the strict sacramental rules of the church. In fact, many displayed exemplary conduct in family, social and work contexts. These men, at one time inhabiting a rather low level in the social hierarchy, had become pillars of the community, achieving positions of prominence and respect. No doubt, impressive conversion experiences also occur within religious environments that do not use hallucinogens, but the question remains: What might the value be of having a pharmacologically active catalyst, in this case one with an extensive history of safe use by the indigenous peoples of South America? Could a person with a serious drug addiction or who engages in antisocial behaviors be "transformed" through a drug-induced mystical experience? There are many sociological, anthropological and psychological studies suggesting that certain drugs—primarily hallucinogens—when taken in a properly structured context (be it a religious group or a psychotherapeutic environment) can promote healing and positive changes in a person's life.

In 1987, the Brazilian government declared ayahuasca a legal substance when used within the context of religious practice, thus becoming the first modern nation to allow the spiritual use of plant hallucinogens by its non-indigenous inhabitants. This extraordinary precedent may allow other countries to reconsider the rich potentials that hallucinogens may hold.

Drug Abuse and Prevention

There is a dark side, though, to the use of hallucinogens. Immature individuals often have the reckless misperception that these are nothing more than recreational drugs, unaware that they may encounter unwelcome and disturbing states of mind. This can lead unsuspecting users to additional dangers, bringing upon themselves realms of ever increasing chaos, confusion and terror. Such foolish tampering with hallucinogens may leave the sorry traveler with persistent states of existential anxiety and despair. The message is clear: To approach this path without proper appreciation of the essential safeguards may lead to serious damage. Unfortunately, there are still too many young and unwary individuals who continue to place themselves at risk.

Preventing hallucinogen use among adolescents and young adults has been at the heart of American drug policy, but the policy seems to have failed. Stalwarts of the model will point out that a modest decline in adolescent marijuana use has occurred—from approximately 60 percent to 50 percent over the past twenty years—but this can hardly be called a success. In addition, the constant abuse of alcohol also remains unchecked: Recent surveys show that 30 percent of college age youth engage in frequent binge drinking, in which an individual consumes at least five alcoholic beverages at a single setting. Why then, with billions of dollars invested in our antidrug programs, do so many people continue to abuse alcohol, as well as other dangerous drugs like methamphetamine, cocaine, heroin and phencyclidine (PCP)?

Adolescence is a developmental period of tremendous change, a time of transition from the relative dependence of childhood to the increasing autonomy and responsibility of adulthood. This phase of adolescence is often a period of considerable stress and insecurity, and thus many young people experiment with a variety of drugs in an attempt to escape their painful and discordant feelings. But the drug- and alcohol-induced euphoria is deceptive, for the habitual flight from life's problems culminates in the failure to acquire the developmental task necessary for greater psychological health. Furthermore, the chronic and compulsive use of powerful mood altering substances has a dulling effect upon the cognitive functioning of the brain. Substance abuse often leads to a lack of mental clarity about one's self, one's goals and one's relationships with others. Repetitive use of drugs and alcohol may also lead to a progressive deterioration of drive and motivation, leaving a person feeling apathetic toward life, and may lead to chronic anxiety and depression, accentuating underlying personality problems and disorders. Intensified degrees of loneliness and isolation, along with pronounced feelings of hopelessness and helplessness, perpetuate the need for further drug-induced refuge and escape. As the process intensifies, self-esteem progressively deteriorates, which places the adolescent at greater risk for dangerous and potentially lethal behavior, including suicide.

Other young adults, in contrast to the chronic or compulsive user, do not seem to suffer from their intermittent or brief experimentation with psychoactive substances. Recent research suggests that the difference lies in the presence or absence of serious underlying psychiatric disorders. The vulnerable novice who has poor coping skills (and who has often been raised in a family environment filled with severe dysfunctional behavior) is more likely to become dependent upon the use of drugs to alleviate psychological suffering. This type of individual will often return again and again to alcohol or drugs as a vehicle for escape. It is essential to identify those who are at greatest risk for progressing from casual use to chronic dependence. Preexisting clinical depression, early experimentation with drugs and alcohol and family psychopathology are three clear indicators of an adolescent who is at risk. Early identification and treatment of these young individuals is critical if we are to effectively redirect such self-destructive behavior.

Alternative perspectives may also be illuminating. A review of the anthropological literature reveals that psychoactive substances have played an important role in human culture dating back to the earliest evidence of human existence. In tribal societies, the incorporation of plant hallucinogens in group or individual initiation rites was widespread. In such contexts, these plant drugs were accepted as being of sacred origin and were treated with awe and reverence. Because of limited supply, the powerful psychotropic plants were under control of adult authority and reserved solely for ritual use. Many tribal groups administered these substances to their youth in pubertal rites of initiation, always under the supervision of the elders of the community. The purpose of this powerful experience was to create a symbolic death of the child followed by emergence into initiatory rebirth of the new adult identity. In contemporary Western culture, however, there is an utter lack of such initiatory and transitional rites and traditions with consequent disregard of safeguards and accentuation of dangers. What was once a sacred and reverent utilization of psychoactive substances among tribal peoples has devolved into the profaned and pathological phenomenon we now define as drug abuse.

To begin to get a better grasp on the epidemic problem of drug misuse and abuse, our public educational models must also be reexamined. Should we heighten vigilance and increase punishments, or should we overhaul our current drug policies and programs and focus more on treatment? Judging from the unchecked and persistent use of alcohol and illicit substances, the dominant *Just Say No* model has not proved to be adequate. One solution is to provide accurate information on how to reduce the potential for drug-induced harm. A drug education program based on a model of *Just Tell The Truth* may be far more effective. Young people want and need to know the truth, and we should be able to offer an education that honestly describes the full range of effects that various drugs cause. By providing alternative perspectives and paradigms, we will enable our young people to make better choices and to incur less risk. By identifying rules of safety and support, more people, young and old, are likely to make decisions based on self-protection and self-preservation. If the true priority is to protect our young from injury, then we need to learn from the past and stop repeating the same mistakes, and in the process create a healthier and more humane world for tomorrow.

About This Anthology

This book has its origins in a series of discussions I had five years ago with publisher Jeremy Tarcher on a topic of mutual interest, the hallucinogens and their implications to the future of our society. Originally, we explored compiling a collection of firsthand accounts from individuals who were notable both for their level of accomplishment in the world and for their attribution of much of their success to transformative experiences they had had with hallucinogens during critical periods of their lives. Although we found no difficulty in attracting qualified individuals willing to submit a contribution to the collection, virtually all came with the stipulation that we publish the accounts under a pseudonym. As the goal of such a project was for respected members of our society to speak openly about these valuable experiences, it would have run counter to the purpose of the book to conceal the identities of contributors.

An alternative plan we chose was to compile a collection of some of the best writing on the issue of hallucinogens published over the last ten years. In spite of the veil of silence that has fallen over the topic during the last quarter-century, a modest but steady stream of excellent essays has been published in the lay literature, attesting to the persistence of serious thought and discussion of the issue. Consequently, selections were chosen from the most engaging articles published in the decade of the nineties, addressing a broad range of perspectives. This anthology contains sixteen essays by leading investigators and theorists in the fields of science, medicine, psychology, anthropology and religious studies. They have been selected in order to illustrate the many dimensions of the hallucinogen experience and their implications to the future development of society. From personal memoirs to sophisticated research, these essays will hopefully encourage further study and more careful reflection regarding the uses and abuses of these remarkable drugs.

—Charles S. Grob, M.D.
Irvine, California
January 15, 2001

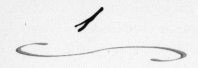

A Conversation
with Albert
Hofmann

Charles S. Grob, M.D.

*In November 1996, I interviewed Albert Hofmann near his home in
Basel, Switzerland. At the age of ninety, Dr. Hofmann appeared robust
and healthy. Excerpts from this interview cover a variety of issues ranging
from his views on the essential lessons learned from the mistakes of the
past to how his personal encounters with hallucinogens resonated with
his early experiences in nature. Grasping the traps and potential risks of
taking these substances within purely recreational contexts, he frames
the case for understanding the spiritual construct within which native
peoples utilized their plant hallucinogen sacraments. Through the adaptation of a transpersonal vision of psychiatry, Hofmann presents his vision of how sacred medicines may be successfully incorporated into our
future society.*

CG: Dr. Hofmann, thank you for speaking with me. I would like to
tape-record our discussion, with the understanding that you will be pro-

vided a transcript for review and approval before publication. I would first like to ask how old are you currently, and how is your health?

AH: I am 90 years old, and I am feeling very fit. I had knee surgery last month, but am now doing very well. The rehabilitation hospital has provided excellent physical therapies for my knee, and I am almost ready to go home to Rittematte. I am in very good condition, and swim in the indoor pool every day. I will miss the swimming, but I am looking forward to going home soon.

CG: I would like to speak with you about your views on psychedelic drugs. To start with, do you believe it is possible to reestablish psychedelic research as a respectable scientific field?

AH: I think there are many good signs. After years of silence, there have recently been some investigations in Switzerland and Germany, and also in the United States. We had a meeting in Heidelberg last year [European College for the Study of Consciousness], and there were many good presentations. In Heidelberg I enjoyed meeting with Rick Doblin [of MAPS] and Professor Nichols [of the Heffter Research Institute], and I think both of their organizations are doing fine work. Their approach appears to be quite different than that of some of their predecessors from several decades ago.

CG: Are you referring to Dr. Leary?

AH: Yes. I was visited by Timothy Leary when he was living in Switzerland many years ago. He was a very intelligent man, and quite charming. I enjoyed our conversations very much. However, he also had a need for too much attention. He enjoyed being provocative, and that shifted the focus from what should have been the essential issue. It is unfortunate, but for many years these drugs became taboo. Hopefully, these same problems from the sixties will not be repeated.

CG: From the vantage point of where we are now, in the late 1990s, what implications do psychedelic drugs have to the field of psychiatry?

AH: I believe that shortly after LSD was discovered, it was recognized as being of great value to psychoanalysis and psychiatry. It was not considered to be an escape. It was a very important discovery at that time, and for fifteen years it could be used legally in psychiatric treatment and for scientific study in humans. During this time, Delysid, the name I gave to LSD, was used safely, and was the subject of thousands of publications in the professional literature. Actually, just last week, I had visitors from the Albert Hofmann Foundation, to whom I gave all of the original documentation, which had been stored at the Sandoz Laboratories. This early work was very well documented, and shows how well research with LSD went until it became part of the drug scene in the 1960s. So, from originally being part of the therapeutic pharmacopeia, LSD became a drug of the street and inevitably it was made illegal. Because of this reputation, it became unavailable to the medical field, and so the research, which had been very open, was stopped. Now it appears that this research may start again. The importance of such investigations appears to be recognized by the health authorities, and so it is my hope that finally the prohibition is coming to an end, and the medical field can return to the explorations which were forced to stop thirty years ago.

CG: What recommendations would you give to researchers now who want to work with these substances?

AH: When LSD was distributed legally by Sandoz, there was a little brochure which was given together with the Delysid, which explained how LSD could be used. As an aid to psychoanalysis and psychotherapy, and also as a means for psychiatrists themselves to experience these extraordinary states of mind. It was specifically stated on the package insert that the psychiatrist who was interested in using Delysid should first test it on himself.

CG: So, you would say that it is very important that the researcher, the psychiatrist, know firsthand the psychedelic experience?

AH: Absolutely, absolutely. Before it can be used in clinical work, it must most definitely be taken by the psychiatrist. From the very first reports and guidelines written for LSD, this was clearly stated. And this remains of utmost importance today.

CG: Are there lessons we can learn from the past insofar as what went wrong with the research, why it was stopped, that we should be attentive to, so mistakes are not repeated?

AH: Yes, if it would be possible to stop their improper use, their misuse, then I think it would be possible to dispense them for medical use. But as long as they continue to be misused, and as long as people fail to truly understand psychedelics and continue to use them as pleasure drugs and fail to appreciate the very deep, deep, psychic experiences they may induce, then their medical use will be held back. Their use on the streets has been a problem for more than thirty years. On the streets the drugs are misunderstood, and accidents occur. This makes it very difficult for the health authorities to change their policies and allow medical use. And although it should be possible to convince the health authorities that in responsible hands psychedelics could be used safely in the medical field, their use on the streets continues to make it very hard for the health authorities to agree.

CG: It appears that young people are once again becoming interested in psychedelics and MDMA. We also have this new phenomenon of the rave, where young people take substances like MDMA and dance all night. What is your view on why these young people seek out such experiences? How can we respond to what they are doing?

AH: This is a very, very deep problem of our time in that we no longer have a religious basis in our lives. Even with religion, with the churches, they are no longer convincing with their dogma. And people need a deep spiritual foundation for their lives. In older times it was religion, with its dogmas, which people believed in, but today those dogmas no longer work. We cannot believe things which we know are not possible, that are not real. We must go on the basis of what we know, that everybody can experience. On this basis, you must find the entrance to the spiritual world. Because many young people are looking for meaningful experiences, they are looking for this thing which is the opposite of the material world. Not all young people are looking for money and power. Some are looking for a happiness and satisfaction which is of the spiritual world, not the materialistic world. They are looking, but there are no sanctioned paths. And, of course, one of the ways young people are using is with psychedelic drugs.

CG: What would you say to young people?

AH: What I would say would most certainly be: Open your eyes! The doors of perception must be opened. That means these young people must learn by their own experience, to see the world as it was before human be-ings were on this planet. That is the real problem today, that people live in towns and cities, where everything is dead. This material world, made by humans, is a dead world, and will disappear and die. I would tell the young people to go out into the countryside, go to the meadow, go to the garden, go to the woods. This is a world of nature to which we belong, absolutely. It is the circle of life, of which we are an integral part. Open your eyes, and see the browns and greens of the earth, and the light which is the essence of nature. The young need to become aware of this circle of life, and real-ize that it is possible to experience the beauty and deep meaning which is at the core of our relation to nature.

CG: When did you first acquire this visionary appreciation of nature?

AH: When I was a young boy, I had many opportunities to walk through the countryside. I had profound and visionary encounters with na-ture, and this was long before I conducted my initial experiments with LSD. Indeed, my first experiences with LSD were very reminiscent of these early mystical encounters I had had as a child in nature. So, you see that it is even possible to have these experiences without drugs. But many people are blocked, without an inborn faculty to realize beauty, and it is these people who may need a psychedelic in order to have a visionary ex-perience of nature.

CG: How do we reconcile this visionary experience with religion and with scientific truth?

AH: It is important to have the experience directly. Aldous Huxley taught us not to simply believe the words, but to have the experience our-selves. This is why the different forms of religion are no longer adequate. They are simply words, words, words, without the direct experience of what it is the words represent. We are now at a phase of human develop-ment where we have accumulated an enormous amount of knowledge through scientific research in the material world. This is very important knowledge, but it must be integrated. What science has brought to light is true, absolutely true. But this is only one part, only one side of our exis-tence, that of the material world. We have a body, and matter gets older and changes, so therefore as far as our having a body, we must die. But the spiritual world, of course, is eternal, but only insofar as it exists in the moment. It is important that we realize this enormous difference between these two sides of our lives. The material world is the world of our body, but the material world is also where man has made all of these scientific and technological discoveries. We must see, then, that science and technology are based on natural laws. But we must also accept that the material world is only the manifestation of the spiritual world. And if we attempt to manifest something, we will have to make use of the material world. For you and I to speak with one another, we must have tongues, we must have air and so forth. All of this is of the material world. If we were to read about spiritual things, it is only words. We must have the experience directly. And the experience occurs only by opening the mind, and opening all of our senses. Those doors of perception must be cleansed. And if the experience does not come spontaneously, on its own, then we may make use of what Huxley calls a gratuitous grace. This may take the form of psychedelic drugs, or perhaps without drugs through a discipline like yoga. But what is of greatest importance is that we have personal experience. Not words, not beliefs, but experience.

CG: Projecting into the future, do you envision that there may be an accepted role within Euro-American culture for psychedelics?

AH: Absolutely! I am convinced that the importance of psychedelics will be recognized. The pathway for this is through psychiatry, but not the psychoanalytic psychiatry of Freud and not the limited scope of modern biological psychiatry. Rather, it will occur through the new field of transpersonal psychiatry. This transpersonal view takes into account both the material world, including our body, as well as the spiritual world. It recognizes that we are simultaneously part of the material and the spiritual worlds. What fits with the concept of transpersonal psychiatry is that we open our doors of perception. What transpersonal psychiatry tries to give us is a recipe for gaining entrance into the spiritual world. This fits exactly with the results of psychedelics. It stimulates your senses. It opens your perception for your own experience. How this phenomenon affects our existence in the material world can be understood through scientific research, and how we can integrate this knowledge with our spiritual selves can be achieved through the transpersonal path.

CG: Dr. Hofmann, you have lived through two World Wars and a Cold War. When you look ahead into the future of mankind, are you hopeful or not?

AH: I am hopeful for the long distant future, but for the near future I am terribly, terribly pessimistic. I believe that what is occurring in the material world is a reflection of the spiritual state of mankind. I fear that many terrible things will occur around the world, because mankind is in spiritual crisis. But I hope that over time mankind will learn, finally learn, and that there will be hope. I just re-read the twelve lectures Aldous Huxley gave in San Francisco in 1959, called The Human Situation. I think that everything that we are concerned about today, about the ego, consciousness, the survival of mankind, it can all be read in this book. I would like to recommend it. Everything we are now trying to say, the ideas we are formulating, has been discussed by Huxley.

CG: What can we learn from the so-called primitive cultures who used psychedelic substances as part of their religious practices?

AH: I think the most important thing is that they use it in a religious framework and we don't. We must learn from them, we must identify the right structures, we must find new uses. I could imagine that it may be possible to create meditation centers for psychedelic use in natural surroundings, where teachers could have experiences and train to become adepts. I perceive this as being possible, but first psychedelics will have to become available to medicine and psychiatry. And then it should be made available for such spiritual centers. Basically, all that we need to know we can learn from how the primitive people use psychedelics as sacraments, in a religious framework. We need such centers, but we also need the psychiatrists. These psychiatrists must become the Shamans of our times. Then I think we will be ready to move towards this kind of psychopharmacopeia.

CG: Back in the sixties many people became frightened of LSD and other psychedelics, including many psychiatrists. Why was that?

AH: They did not use it the right way, and they did not have the right conditions. So, they were not adequately prepared for it. It is such a delicate and deep experience, if used the right way. But remember, the more powerful the instrument, the more the chance of damage occurring if it is not used properly. And back at that time, there were unfortunately many occasions where psychedelics were not treated with proper respect, and used in the wrong way, and consequently caused injury. That is the great tragedy, that these valuable medicines were not always respected and not always understood. So, the psychedelics came to be feared, and were taken out of the hands of responsible investigators and psychiatrists. It was a great loss for medicine and psychiatry, and for mankind. Hopefully, it is not too late to learn from these mistakes, and to demonstrate the proper and respectful way psychedelics should be used.

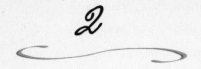

The Role of
Psychoactive
Plant Medicines

Ralph Metzner, Ph.D.

Veteran hallucinogen researcher Ralph Metzner has explored the many cultural contexts within which psychoactive plant medicines have been used throughout history. Contrasting with modern society's chronic incapacity to successfully integrate hallucinogens, Dr. Metzner examines how indigenous healers access a paradigm effectively incorporating religious, medicinal and psychotherapeutic dimensions. A professor of psychology at the California Institute of Integral Studies, Ralph Metzner shares the insights he accrued over four decades of active investigation in the field.

THERE IS A QUESTION that had troubled me, and no doubt others, since the heyday of psychedelic research in the 1960s, when many groups and individuals were preoccupied with the problem of assimilating new and powerful mind-altering substances into Western society. The question, simply stated, was this: Why did the American Indians succeed in integrating the use of peyote into their culture, including its legal use as a

sacrament to this day, when those interested in pursuing consciousness research with drugs in the dominant white culture succeeded only in having
the entire field made taboo to research and any use of the substances
deemed a criminal offense punishable by imprisonment? The use of peyote spread from Mexico to the North American Indian tribes in the latter
half of the nineteenth century and has found acceptance as a sacrament in
the ceremonies of the Native American Church. It is recognized as one
kind of religious ritual that some of the tribes practice; and it is acknowledged by sociologists for its role as an antidote for alcohol abuse.

This intriguing puzzle in ethnopsychology and social history was relevant to me, since I was one of the psychedelic researchers who saw the
enormous transformative potentials of "consciousness expanding" drugs,
as we called them, and were eager to continue the research into their psychological significance. It would be fair to state that none of the early explorers in this field, in the fifties and early sixties, had any inkling of the
social turmoil that was to come or of the vehemence of the legal-political
reaction. Certainly Albert Hofmann, the Swiss chemist who discovered
LSD—the epitome of the cautious, conservative scientist—has testified to
his dismay and concern over the proliferation of patterns of abuse of what
he so poignantly called his "problem child" (Sorgenkind).

Thus resulted the strange paradox that substances regarded as a social
evil and a law enforcement problem in the mainstream dominant culture
are the sacrament of one particular subculture within that larger society.
Since the Native American subcultures are older and ecologically more sophisticated cultures than the European white culture that attempted to
absorb or eliminate it, and since many sensitive individuals have long argued that we should be learning from the Indians, not exterminating them,
the examination of the question I have posed could lead to highly interesting conclusions. The answer to the ethnopsychological puzzle became
clear to me only after I started observing and participating in a number of
other American Indian ceremonies that did not involve the use of peyote,
such as a healing-singing circle, a sweat lodge, and a spirit dance. I noted
what many ethnologists have reported—that these ceremonies were simultaneously religious, medicinal, and psychotherapeutic. The sweat lodge,

like the peyote ritual, is regarded as a sacred ceremony, as a form of worship of the Creator; they are also both seen and practiced as a form of physical healing, and they are performed for solving personal and collective
psychological problems. Thus it was natural for those tribes that took up
peyote to add this medium to the others with which they were already familiar, as a ceremony that expressed and reinforced the integration of body,
mind, and spirit.

In the dominant white society, by contrast, medicine, psychology, and
religious spirituality are separated by seemingly insurmountable paradigm
differences. The medical, psychological, and religious professions and
established groups each separately considered the phenomenon of psychedelic drugs and were much too frightened by the unpredictable transformations of perception and worldview that they seemed to trigger. The
dominant society's reaction was fear, followed by total prohibition, even of
further research. None of the three established professions wanted these
consciousness-expanding instruments, and neither did they want anyone
else to be able to use them of their own free choice. The implicit assumption was (and is) that people are too ignorant and gullible to be able to make
reasoned, informed choices as to how to treat their illnesses, solve their
psychological problems, or practice their religion. The fragmented condition of our whole society is mirrored back to us through these reactions.

For the Native Americans, on the other hand, healing, worship, and problem solving are all subsumed in the one way, which is the way of the Great
Spirit, the way of Mother Earth, the traditional way. The integrative understanding given in the peyote visions is not feared, but accepted and respected. Here the implicit assumption is that everyone has the capability,
indeed the responsibility, to attune themselves to higher spiritual sources
of knowledge and healing—and the purpose of ceremony, with or without
medicinal substances, is regarded as a facilitator of such attunement.

Psychedelics as Sacrament or Recreation

Several observers, for example, Andrew Weil, have pointed out the historical pattern that as Western colonial society adopted psychoactive plant

or food substances from native cultures, the use of such psychoactive materials devolved from sacramental to recreational. Tobacco was historically
regarded as a sacred or power plant by Indians of North, Central, and South
America and is still so regarded by Native Americans. In white Western
culture, and in countries influenced by this dominant culture, however,
cigarette smoking is obviously recreational and has become a major public
health problem. The coca plant, as grown and used by the Andean Indian
tribes, was treated as a divinity, Mama Coca, and valued for its health-
maintaining properties. The concentrated extract cocaine, on the other
hand, is purely a recreational drug, and its indiscriminate use as such
causes numerous health problems. In this, and other instances, desecra-
tion of the plant drug has been accompanied by criminalization. Coffee is
another example. Apparently first discovered and used by Islamic Sufis,
who valued its stimulant properties for long nights of prayer and meditation, it became a fashionable recreational drink in European society in
the seventeenth century and was even banned for a while as being too dangerous. And cannabis, used by some sects of Hindu Tantrism as an amplifier of visualization and meditation, has become the epitome of the
recreational "high."

Since sacramental healing plants were so rapidly and completely profaned upon being adopted by the West's increasingly materialistic culture,
it is not surprising that newly discovered synthetic psychoactive drugs have
generally been very quickly categorized as either recreational or narcotic—
even those, like the psychedelics, whose effects are the opposite of narcotic ("sleep inducing"). Concomitantly, as the indiscriminate, excessive,
nonsacramental use of psychoactive plants and newly synthesized analogues spread, so did patterns of abuse and dependence. Predictably, established society reacted with prohibitions, which in turn spawned organized
crime activities. This took place in spite of the fact that many of the original discoverers of the new synthetic psychedelics, such as Albert Hofmann
and Alexander Shulgin, are individuals of deep spiritual integrity. Neither
their efforts nor those of such philosophers as Aldous Huxley, Alan Watts,
and Huston Smith or psychologists such as Timothy Leary and Richard

Alpert, to advocate a sacred and respectful attitude toward these substances, were able to prevent the same profanation.

The newly discovered phenethylamine psychedelic (also called empathogenic—"empathy generating") MDMA provides an instructive example of this phenomenon. Two patterns of use seem to have become established during the seventies. Some psychotherapists and spiritually inclined individuals began to explore its possible applications as a therapeutic adjuvant and as an amplifier of spiritual practice. Another, much larger group of people began using it for recreational purposes, as a social "high" comparable in some respects to cocaine. Its irresponsible and widespread use in this second category by increasing numbers of people understandably made the medical and law enforcement authorities nervous. The predictable reaction occurred. MDMA was classified as a Schedule I drug in the United States, which puts it in the same group as heroin, cannabis, and LSD—making it a criminal offense to make, use, or sell the substance and sending a clearly understood off-limits signal to pharmaceutical and medical researchers.

After Albert Hofmann had identified psilocybin as the psychoactive ingredient in the Mexican magic mushroom that the Aztecs called *teonanacatl,* he took some of the synthesized psilocybin to the Mazatec shamaness Maria Sabina, to obtain her assessment of how closely the synthesized ingredient resembled the natural product. In doing so, he was following the appropriate path of acknowledging the primacy of the botanical over the synthetic. It has been suggested that for every one of the important synthetic psychedelics there is a natural plant that has the same ingredients and that perhaps it should be our research strategy to find the botanical "host" for the psychedelics emerging from the laboratory. Research on the shamanic use of the hallucinogenic morning glory seeds called *ololiuhqui* in ancient Mexico, which contain LSD analogues, has allowed us a deeper understanding of the possible uses of this substance.

If Gordon Wasson, Albert Hofmann, and Carl Ruck are correct in their proposal that an LSD-like ergot-derived beverage was used as the initiatory sacrament in Eleusis, the implications are profound. According to Rupert

Sheldrake's theory of morphogenetic fields, rituals, like any patterned activity, gain their power through precise repetition of all the elements. One could suppose that by regrowing or rehybridizing this particular plant, as it was used in ancient times, we could "tune in" to and reactivate the morphogenetic field of the Eleusinian Mysteries, the ancient world's most awe-inspiring mystical ritual.

There is no inherent reason why sacramental use and recreational use of a substance in moderation cannot coexist. In fact, among Native Americans, tobacco often plays this dual role; after a sacred pipe ritual with tobacco and other herbs, participants may smoke cigarettes to relax. We know the sacramental use of wine in the Catholic Communion rite, and we certainly know the recreational use of wine. We are able to keep the two contexts separate, and we are also able to recognize when recreational use becomes dependence and abuse. One could envision a similar sophistication developing with regard to psychoactive plant products. There could be recognized sacramental and therapeutic applications, and certain patterns of use might develop that are more playful, exploratory, and hedonistic— and yet contained within a reasonable and acceptable social framework that minimizes harm. The abuse of a drug in such a rational and sensible system would not be a function of who uses it, or where it originated, or its chemical classification—but rather the behavioral consequences of the drug user. Someone becomes recognized as an alcoholic, that is, an abuser of alcohol, when his or her interpersonal and social relationships are noticeably impaired. There should be no difficulty in establishing similar abuse criteria for other psychoactive drugs.

Psychedelics as Gnostic Catalysts

In 1968, in an article called "On the Evolutionary Significance of Psychedelics," I suggested that the findings of LSD research in the areas of psychology, religion, and the arts could be considered in the context of the evolution of consciousness. "If LSD expands consciousness and if, as is widely believed, further evolution will take the form of an increase in consciousness, then can we not regard LSD as a possible *evolutionary instru-*

ment? . . . Here is a device which, by altering the chemical composition of
the cerebro-sensory information processing medium, temporarily inacti-
vates the screening-programs, the genetic and cultural filters, which dom-
inate in a completely unnoticed way our usual perceptions of the world."
From the perspective of almost thirty years' experience and reflection, I
would now extend and amplify this statement in two ways:

1. The evolution of consciousness is a transformational process that
   consists primarily in gaining insight and understanding, or gnosis.
2. The acceleration of this process by molecular catalysts not only is
   a consequence of new chemical discoveries but also is an integral
   component of traditional systems of transformation, including
   shamanism, alchemy, and yoga.

In the field of consciousness research, the "set-and-setting hypothesis,"
which was first formulated by Timothy Leary in the early sixties, helps us
understand psychoactive drugs and plants as one class of triggers within a
whole range of possible catalysts of altered states. The theory states that
the content of a psychedelic experience is a function of the set (intention,
attitude, personality, mood) and the setting (interpersonal, social, and environmental) and that the drug functions as a kind of trigger, or catalyst, or
nonspecific amplifier or sensitizer. The hypothesis can be applied to the
understanding of any altered state of consciousness, when we recognize
that other kinds of stimuli can be triggers—for example, hypnotic induction, meditation techniques, mantra, sound or music, breathing, sensory
isolation, movement, sex, natural landscapes, a near-death experience, and
the like.

An important clarification results from keeping in mind the distinction
between a state (of consciousness) and a psychological trait, between state
changes and trait changes. For example, psychologists distinguish between
state anxiety and trait anxiety. William James, in his classic *Varieties of Religious Experience,* discussed this question in terms of whether a religious
or conversion experience would necessarily lead to more "saintliness,"
more enlightened traits. This distinction is crucial to the assessment of the

value or significance of drug-induced altered states. Only by attending to both the state changes (visions, insights, feelings) and the long-term consequences, or behavioral or trait changes, can a comprehensive understanding of these phenomena be attained.

Having an insight is not the same as being able to apply that insight. There is no inherent connection between a mystical experience of oneness and the expression or manifestation of that oneness in the affairs of everyday life. This point is perhaps obvious, and yet it is frequently overlooked by those who argue, on principle, that a drug cannot induce a genuine mystical experience or play any role in spiritual life. The internal factors of *set,* including preparation, expectation, and intention, are the determinants of whether a given experience is authentically religious. Equally, intention is crucial to the question of whether an altered state results in any lasting personality changes. Intention is the bridge from the ordinary or "consensus reality" state to the state of heightened consciousness; and it also provides a bridge from that heightened state back to ordinary reality.

This model allows us to understand how the same drug(s) could be claimed by some to lead to nirvana or religious vision and in others (for example, Charles Manson) could lead to perverse and sadistic violence. The drug is only a tool, a catalyst, to attain certain altered states; which altered states depend on the intention. Furthermore, even where the drug-induced state is benign and expansive, whether it leads to long-lasting positive changes is also a matter of intention or mind-set.

The drug indeed seems to reveal or release something that is *in* the person. This is the factor implied in the term *psychedelic,* which means "mind manifesting." An alternate term that has been proposed is *entheogenic,* "releasing (or generating) the deity within." My reservation about this term is that it might convey the misleading idea that the divinity within is "generated" in these states. To the contrary, most people realize in these states that the divine within *is* the generator, the source of life energy, the awakening and healing power. For someone whose conscious intention is a psychospiritual transformation, the psychedelic *can* be a catalyst that reveals and releases insight or knowledge from higher aspects of our being. This is,

I believe, what is meant by *gnosis*—sacred knowledge, insight concerning the fundamental spiritual realities of the universe in general, and one's individual destiny in particular.

The potential of psychedelic drugs to act as catalysts to a transformation into gnosis, or direct, ongoing awareness of divine reality, even if only in a small number of people, would seem to be of the utmost significance. Traditionally, the number of individuals who have had mystical experiences has been very small; the number of those who have been able to make practical applications of such experiences has probably been even smaller. Thus, the discovery of psychedelics, in facilitating such experiences and processes, could be regarded as one very important factor in a general spiritual awakening of collective human consciousness. Other factors that could be mentioned in this connection are the revolutionary paradigm shifts in the physical and biological sciences, the burgeoning interest in Eastern philosophies and spiritual disciplines, and the growing awareness of the multicultural oneness of the human family brought about by the global communications networks.

Psychedelics in Traditional Systems of Transformation

In earlier writings I emphasized the newness of psychedelic drugs and the unimaginable potentials to be realized by their constructive application. I viewed them as first products of a new technology, oriented toward the human spirit. I still appreciate the potential role of the new synthetic psychedelics in consciousness research and perhaps in consciousness evolution. My views have changed somewhat, however, under the influence of the discoveries and writings of cultural anthropologists and ethnobotanists, who have pointed to the role of mind-altering and visionary botanicals in traditional cultures across the world.

Shamanism

One cannot read the works of R. Gordon Wasson on the Mesoamerican mushroom cults; or the work of Richard E. Schultes on the profusion of hallucinogens in the Amazon region; or the cross-cultural studies of such authors as Michael Harner, Joan Halifax, Peter Furst, and Luis Eduardo Luna; or the cross-culturally oriented medical and psychiatric works of such researchers as Andrew Weil, Claudio Naranjo, and Stanislav Grof; or more personal accounts, such as the writings of Carlos Castaneda, Florinda Donner, the McKenna brothers, or Bruce Lamb's biography of Manuel Cordova, without gaining a strong sense of the pervasiveness of the quest for visions, insights, and nonordinary states of consciousness in the world-wide shamanic traditions. These studies demonstrate incontrovertibly that psychoactive plants are used in many, but by no means all of the shamanic cultures that pursue such states. For this reason I have been led to a view closer to that of aboriginal cultures, a view of humanity in a relationship of co-consciousness, communication, and cooperation with the animal king-dom, the plant kingdom, and the mineral world. In such a worldview, the ingestion of hallucinogenic plant preparations to obtain knowledge—for healing, for prophecy, for communication with spirits, for anticipation of danger, or for understanding the universe—appears as one of the oldest and most highly treasured traditions.

The various shamanic cultures all over the world know a wide variety of means for entering nonordinary realities. Michael Harner has pointed out that "auditory driving" with prolonged drumming is perhaps equally as widespread a technology for entering shamanic states as hallucinogens. In some cultures, the rhythmic hyperventilation produced through certain kinds of chanting may be another form of altered-state trigger. Animal spir-its become guides and allies in shamanic initiation. Plant spirits can be-come "helpers," too, even when the plant is not taken internally by either doctor or patient. Tobacco smoke is used as a purifier as well as a support to prayer. Crystals are used to focus energy for seeing and healing. There is attunement, through prayer and meditation, with deities and spirits of the land, the four directions, the elements, the Creator Spirit. The knowl-edge obtained from other states and other worlds is used to improve the way we live in this world. The use of hallucinogenic plants is part of an in-tegrated complex of interrelationships among nature, spirit, and human consciousness.

Thus it seems to me that the lessons we are to learn from these consciousness-expanding plants in shamanism have to do not only with the recognition of other dimensions of the human psyche but also with a radically different worldview—a worldview that has been maintained in the beliefs, practices, and rituals of shamanic cultures and almost totally forgotten or suppressed by the materialist culture of the modern age. There is, of course, a certain delightful irony in the fact that it has taken a material substance to awaken the sleeping consciousness of so many of our contemporaries to the reality of nonmaterial energies, forms, and beings.

Alchemy

In discussing alchemy as the second of the three traditional systems of consciousness transformation mentioned earlier, I would emphasize first that we have only the minutest shreds of evidence that ingestion of hallucinogens played any part in the European alchemical tradition. The use of solanaceous (nightshades) hallucinogens in European witchcraft, which is related to both shamanism and alchemy, has been documented by Harner. Likewise, in Chinese Taoist alchemy, the use of botanical and mineral preparations to induce spirit flight and other kinds of altered states, has been discussed by Michel Strickmann. A complete account of the role of hallucinogens in alchemy has not as yet been written. Possibly, our ignorance in this field is still a consequence of intentional secrecy on the part of the alchemical writers.

Mircea Eliade, in his book *The Forge and the Crucible,* made a strong case for the historical derivation of alchemy from early Bronze Age and Iron Age metallurgy, mining, and smithing rites and practices. One could argue that alchemy is one form of shamanism—the shamanism of those who worked with minerals and metals, the makers of tools and weapons. Many of the concerns and interests of the alchemists parallel shamanic themes. There is the strong interest in purification and healing, in discovering or making a "tincture" or "elixir" that will impart health and longevity. There are visions and encounters with animal spirits, some clearly from the imaginal realms. There are stories and visions of divine and semidivine figures, often personified as the deities of classical mythology. There is the recognition of the sacredness, the animating spirit, of all matter. And there is the integrated worldview, which sees spirituality, religion, health and illness, human beings, and the natural world and its elements all interrelated in a totality.

It is true that there does not seem to be the equivalent of a shamanic journey in alchemy, no clear indication of an altered state of consciousness in which visions or power or healing abilities are attained. It appears to me, however, that the alchemical equivalent of the shamanic journey is the opus, the "work," the experiment with its various operations, such as *solutio, sublimatio, mortificatio,* and the like. The focus would seem to be more on the long-term personality and physical changes that the alchemical initiate has to undergo, just like the shaman in training. The operations in alchemy were meditative rituals, during which visions might be seen in the retort or furnace, and interior psychophysiological state changes triggered by the empathic observation of chemical processes.

Furthermore, R. J. Stewart has argued that in the Western tradition of magic and alchemy, which has roots in pre-Christian Celtic mythology and beliefs and of which traces can still be found in folklore, ballads, popular songs, and nursery rhymes, the central transformative experience was the Underworld journey. This Underworld or "otherworld" initiation involved taking a "journey" into other realms, encounters with animal and spirit beings, attunement with the land and the ancestors, meditative rituals centering around the tree-of-life symbolism, and other features that place this tradition clearly in the ancient stream of shamanic lore found in all parts of the globe.

Yoga

Turning now to yoga as the third of the traditional systems of evolutionary transformation of consciousness, we need not try to resolve the questions of whether the use of psychoactive plant preparations is a decadent form of yoga, as Eliade seems to believe, or whether the use of hallucinogens was primary, in the Vedic Indian tradition of the soma cult, as Wasson has proposed. Some have suggested that methods of yoga were developed when the psychoactive plant or fungus was no longer available, as an alternative means for attaining visionary states. Suffice it to say that in the Indian yogic traditions, in particular the teachings of Tantra, we have a system of practices for bringing about a transformation of consciousness, with many parallels to shamanic and alchemical ideas.

The use of hallucinogens as an adjunct to yogic practices is known to this day in India, among certain Shaivite sects in particular. Those schools and sects that do not use drugs tend to regard those that do as decadent, as belonging to the so-called left-hand path of Tantra, which also incorporates ritual food and sexuality (*maithuna*) as valid aspects of the yogic practice. Under the influence of nineteenth-century Western occult and theosophical ideas, this left-hand path was equated to "black magic" or "sorcery." In actuality, the designation "left-hand path" derives from the yogic principle that the left side of the body is the feminine, receptive side; thus, the left-hand path is the path of those who worship the Goddess (*Shakti*), as the Tantrics do, and incorporate the experience of body, the delight of the senses, food, and sexuality into their yoga. Thus, as in shamanism and alchemy, we find here a strand of the tradition that involves respect and devotion to the feminine principle, the Mother Goddess, the earth and its fruit, the flesh-and-blood body, and the seeking of ecstatic visionary states.

It is true that the Indian yogic traditions seem not to have the same concern for the natural world of animals, crystals, and plants as is found in shamanism and alchemy. The emphasis is more on various inner and subtle states of consciousness. Nevertheless, there are interesting parallels among the three traditions. The focusing of inner light-fire energy in different centers and organs of the body, as practiced in Agni Yoga and Kundalini Yoga, is similar to the alchemical practice of purification by fire and to shamanic notions of filling the body with light. The Indian alchemical Tantric tradition embraced the concept of *rasa*, which is akin to the European alchemical concept of "tincture" or "elixir." Rasa has internal meanings—feeling, mood, "soul"—and external referents—essence, juice, liquid. *Rasayana* was the path or way of rasa, the way of fluid energy flow, which involves both external and internal essences. As a third parallel, I will only mention the Tibetan Buddhist Vajrayana system, which is a remarkable fu-

sion of Tantric Buddhist ideas with the original Bon shamanism of Tibet—
a system in which the various animal spirits and demons of the shamans
and sorcerers have become transformed into personifications of Buddhist
principles and guardians of the dharma.

Conclusions

It appears incontrovertible that plant (and fungal) hallucinogens played
some role, of unknown extent, in the transformative traditions of shamanism, alchemy, and yoga. If we regard psychotherapy as the modern de-
scendant of these traditional systems, then a similar, if limited, application
of hallucinogens could be made in various aspects of psychotherapy. And
this has, in fact, already occurred, as the various studies of psychedelics in
alcoholism, terminal cancer, obsessional neurosis, depression, and other
conditions testify. It seems likely that these kinds of applications of psychedelics, as adjuncts to psychotherapy, will continue—if not with LSD
and other Schedule I drugs, then with other, newer and perhaps safer psychedelics.

What appears unlikely to me is that this kind of controlled psychiatric
application will ever be enough to satisfy the inclinations and needs of
those individuals who wish to explore psychedelics in their most ancient
role, as tools for seeking visionary states and hidden forms of knowledge.
The fact that the serious use of hallucinogens, outside a psychiatric framework, continues despite severe social and legal sanctions suggests that this
is a kind of individual freedom that is not easy to abolish. It also suggests
that there is a strong need in certain people to reestablish their connections with ancient traditions of knowledge, in which visionary states of
consciousness and exploration of other realities, with or without hallucinogens, were the central concern.

It may be that such a path will always be pursued by only a limited
number of individuals—much as the shamanic, alchemical, and yogic ini-
tiations and practices were pursued by only a few individuals in each society. I find it a hopeful sign that some people, however few, are willing to
explore how to reconnect with these lost sources of knowledge, because,

like many others, I feel that our materialist-technological society, with its fragmented worldview, has largely lost its way and can ill afford to ignore any potential aids to greater knowledge of the human mind. The ecologically balanced and integrative framework of understanding the ancient traditions preserved surely has much to offer us.

Furthermore, it is clear that the visions and insights of the individuals who pursue these paths are visions and insights for the present and the future and not just of historical or anthropological interest. This has always been the pattern: the individual seeks a vision to understand his or her place, or destiny, as a member of the community. The knowledge derived from expanded states of consciousness has been, can be, and needs to be applied to the solution of the staggering problems that confront our species. This is why the discoveries of the mystical chemists and ethnobotanists have immense importance—for the understanding of our past, the awareness of our presence, and the safeguarding of our future.

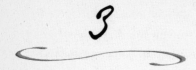

Psychedelic Society

Terence McKenna

A prominent scholar over the past two decades on the phenomenology of the hallucinogen experience has been ethnobotanist Terence McKenna. Together with his brother Dennis, with whom he made valuable contributions to our understanding of psychoactive plants native to the remote Amazon, Terence McKenna has provided challenging perspectives on the implications of the core hallucinogen experience to our fundamental conception of reality. Examining the potential of these substances to act as deconditioning agents, McKenna in this provocative article envisions the transformation of human society.

I WANT TO TALK TONIGHT about the notion of a psychedelic society. When I spoke in Santa Barbara at a psychedelics conference my contact lenses failed me at a critical point in my lecture and I simply had to wing it. Later when I played this tape back I heard the phrase "psychedelic society." I never used it before consciously in a lecture. But because I had said it, and because there had been a ripple of resonance to it from the people there, I began to think about it and this evening I will generally assess what it might mean for us.

When I think of psychedelic society that notion implies creating a society which lives in light of the Mystery of Being. In other words, problems and solutions should be displaced from the central role they have had in social organizations, and Mysteries—*irreducible Mysteries*—should be in their place. In the 1920s the British entomologist J.B.S. Haldane said in an essay, "The universe may not only be stranger than we suppose; it may be stranger than we *can* suppose."

I suggest that as we look back over human history every pinnacle of civilization—whether it be Mayan, or Greco-Roman, or the Sung Dynasty— has believed that it was in possession of an accurate description of the cosmos and of man's relationship to it. This seems to go along with the full flowering of a civilization. But from the point of view of our present civilization we regard all those earlier conceptions as at worst quaint, at best half right. We congratulate ourselves that our civilization at last has its finger on the real description of what is going on.

I think this is an error, and that actually what blinds us, or makes historical progress very difficult, is our lack of awareness that our beliefs have grown obsolete and should be put aside. A psychedelic society would abandon belief systems for direct experience. This is I think much of the problem of the modern dilemma: direct experience has been discounted, and in its place all kinds of belief systems have been erected.

I would prefer a kind of intellectual anarchy where whatever was pragmatically applicable was brought to bear on any situation; where belief was understood as a self-limiting function. Because, you see, if you believe something, you are automatically precluded from believing its opposite; which means that a degree of your human freedom has been forfeited in the act of committing yourself to this belief.

I maintain that it is pointless to have beliefs, because if the universe really is stranger than we suppose, what we need is a return to what in the sixteenth century was called the Baconian method; which means not the elaboration of fantastic thought constructs which explain nature, but merely a phenomenological cataloging of what we experience. Computer

networks and psychedelic drugs and the increased availability of information in the world have actually made possible the evolution of new information states which never existed before. We are processing these new
opportunities at a very slow rate because we are hindered by ideology.

Freudian and Jungian models of the psychedelic experience see it as a
stripping away of resistance revealing hidden and complex emotions, mo-
tives, and belief systems. This notion has been replaced in the last five to
ten years by the shamanic model of hallucinogenic experience. This model
holds that archaic peoples have deputized special members of society to
probe hidden information domains using psychedelic drugs. The information extracted from these domains is then used to guide and direct the
society.

I am interested in this second model. I've spent time in the Amazon and
am familiar with the operational mechanics of shamanism and shamanic
personalities. I believe that the psychedelic experience looms larger even
than the institution of shamanism. We are facing a unique opportunity,
which is the flip side of the global culture crisis.

Our ability to destroy ourselves is the mirror image of our ability to save
ourselves. What is lacking is a clear vision of what should be done. What
should be done is certainly not the accumulation of ever-larger thermonu-
clear arsenals and the promotion of all kinds of primate game-playing—the
sort that Tim Leary is well versed in denouncing. What needs to be done
is that our fundamental ontological conceptions of reality have to be re-
made. We need a new language, and in order to have a new language we
must have a new reality. It's a kind of uroboric equation, or a bootstrap situation. A new reality will generate a new language. A new language will
make a new reality legitimate and a part of this reality.

The psychedelic substances can be conceived of as points of an infor-
mational grid. They provide new perspectives on reality, and when you reconnect all the points of view that you have collected regarding reality then
a reasonably applicable model of reality begins to appear.

I think this reasonably applicable model of reality—what Wittgenstein
called something that is "true enough"—is what we are looking for. The
"true enough" mapping of experience onto theory is what we are looking

for, but experience must be made primary. The language of the self must be made primary.

What I am advocating is that we each take responsibility for the cultural transformation by realizing that it is not something which will be disseminated from the top down. It is something which each of us can contribute to by attempting to live as far into the future as possible. We must get rid of the conceptions of the 40s, the 50s, the 60s, the 70s, the 80s, the 90s. We must transcend the historical moment and become exemplars of humanity at the End of Time.

Those of you who attended my lecture this afternoon concerning time know that I believe that liberation—or let's even say "decency"—as a human quality is a resonance and anticipation of this future perfected state of humanity. We can will the perfect future into being by becoming microcosms of the perfect future, no longer casting blame outward onto institutions or hierarchies of responsibility or control, but realizing the opportunity is here, the responsibility is here, and the two may never be congruent again. The salvation of your immortal soul may depend on what you do with the opportunity life places before you.

So, what do we do with the opportunity? What does it mean to say, in operational terms, "Live as far into the future as you can?" It means taking a position *vis à vis* the emergent hyper-dimensional reality. It does not necessarily mean becoming a psychedelic drug user yourself; but it does mean admitting to the possibility. If you feel the heroic potential within to be one of the experiencers—one of the pioneers—then you know what to do. If on the other hand you feel lost in the abyss—you feel what William Blake called "the falling into eternal death," falling from the spiral of being which connects one incarnation to another—then you orient yourself toward the psychedelic experience as a source of information.

A mirror image of the psychedelic experience has emerged in the integrated hardware and software comprising the computer networks. The Internet and the World Wide Web are, paradoxically enough, a deeply feminizing influence on society. It is in hardware/software development that the unconscious is actually becoming conscious. It is as though we took the Platonic *bon mot*—"If God did not exist, man would invent him"—and said, "If the unconscious did not exist, humanity will invent it in the form of these vast networks that are able to transfer and transform information."

This is, in fact, what we are caught up in: the transforming of information. We have not physically changed in the last forty thousand years. The human type was established well before the end of the last glaciation. Change which previously operated in the biological realm is now operating in the realm of culture. And we are shedding cultural assumptions concerning our vision of the unitary mystery at a faster and faster rate as we try to accommodate ourselves to the unfolding of that mystery which lies ahead of us in time. It is that process which is casting a vast shadow of fatedness back over the entire experience of human history.

Previous to our own era, the only word which could be applied to this force that is bringing people together, causing birth and death, tearing down and erecting civilizations, was God; and it was imagined as a self-conscious force that was leaning into the world like a cat into a fishbowl and making things happen. Now we have a different notion—a notion of a vector system where forces over a large area are oriented toward a very small space and this dense micro-sector of space/time is what history is. It is an inrushing toward what the Buddhists call "the realm of the densely-packed," a transformational realm where the opposites are unified.

History is that realm where the body is finally interiorized and the mind is finally exteriorized. The way I think of the mind is as a fourth dimensional organ of your body. You can't see it because it is in the fourth dimension, but you experience a lower dimensional sectioning of it in the phenomenon of consciousness. But that is only a partial sectioning of it; the way an ellipse is a partial picture of a cone.

The growth of information systems is only a mirroring in masculine hardware of what already exists in nature as a fact. It is up to us to hone our intuitions and to become aware of this preexisting system of communication and wiring so that we can step away from the dualisms that separate us from each other and from the world. We need to realize that there is a gene swarm—not a set of species—on the earth; that half the time you think you are thinking you are actually listening; that ideas are remarkably slippery creatures that are very difficult to trace to their origin; and that we really are one-on-one and all together in a dimension that is not as accessible as you might wish to be congealed (as Joyce comments in *Finnegan's Wake*).

The psychedelics are a red-hot, social/ethical issue precisely because they are deconditioning agents. They will raise doubts in you if you are a Hassidic rabbi, a Marxist anthropologist, or an altar boy because their business is to dissolve belief systems. They do this very well, and then they leave you with the raw datum of experience, what William James called— talking of infantile experience—"a blooming, buzzing confusion."

Out of that you reconstruct the world and you need to understand that this reconstruction is a dialogue where your decisions—the projection of your grammar onto the intellectual space in front of you—is going to gel into a mode of being. We all create our own universe because we are all operating with our own private languages which are only very crudely translatable into any other person's language. There is even a physical analog to this which will further reinforce this notion of our separateness and our uniqueness.

Your picture of the world impinging on your eyes is made of photons. Photons are tiny wave packets so closely circumscribed interjectionally that they can be thought of as particles. That means that every single photon that falls on the back of my eye is different than every single photon that falls on the back of any one of your eyes. This means that I am relying 100% on a different section of the world than any one of you are to get a picture of it. And yet we are sitting here with the naive assumption that our pictures of the world differ only by our perspective within the space of the room.

We have numerous extremely naive assumptions like this built into our thinking. Our most venerable explanatory engines—such as "science"— happen also to be our oldest explanatory engines. Therefore they have built into them the most naive and unexamined assumptions. "Science," for instance, we can demolish in thirty seconds. "Science" tells you that a set of conditions will create a given effect, and that every time that set of conditions is in place that effect will be found to obtain. The only place this happens is in laboratories. Our experience isn't like that. A contact with a person is always different. The experience of making love, having a meal, riding a bus—these things are always different. It is their uniqueness in fact—the uniqueness which pervades all being—that makes it bearable at all. Yet "science" is willing to tell you that the only things worth describing are those phenomena which can be repeatedly triggered. This is because these are the only phenomena which science can describe, and that's the name of the game as far as it is concerned.

But we need to claim our freedom—to take advantage of the tiny moment between immense abysses of unknowability; perhaps death, perhaps other reincarnations, perhaps transitions into other life forms. These things we don't know or understand but in the moment of being human we have a unique opportunity to figure them out. And I have faith that it is possible—sometime, somewhere—to have a conversation. Perhaps no progress would be made until the ninth hour in which reality could be literally pulled to pieces, beyond the point of reconstruction.

There is definitely an anti-humanist tendency in all systems. Ludwig von Bertalanfe, who was the inventor of general systems theory, said, "People are not machines, but in every situation where they are given the choice they will behave like machines." We all fall into patterns. We then hold those patterns ever more tightly. They cannot be violated; and this happens on the thought level.

We are now at the cresting of the historical wave of this kind of uptightness, uptightness that stretches back millennia. I hope we have come to the end of this phase. Whether you buy into my own peculiar, apocalyptarian transformative vision involving 2012, or whether you just can tell by looking around you that the shit may soon hit the fan, I think that we can agree that we have come to some kind of an impasse. What is going to come out of this situation is either going to be a great deal of dislocation in the biosphere, the invalidation of intelligence as an adaptation of biology, and our extinction, or we are going to become—as James Joyce dreamed we could—"man made dirigible"; in other words, the exteriorization of the soul, the interiorization of the body.

In this process, everything is going to be challenged. The very notion of humanness is going to be challenged. We are on the brink, through genetic manipulation of DNA, of taking control of the human form, of being able to extend the notion of art inward into the human body and form. Are we classicists? Shall we each be an Adonis and a Persephone? Or what are we? Are we surrealists? Shall I be a potato, and you a burning giraffe? These are decisions which will have to be faced. I smile as I speak but these are the important questions.

And the vertical gain notion we see in the metaphors applied to psychedelic experience: consciousness expansion, getting high, psychedelic tripping, shamanic flight. It's like the hallucinogens are the feminine, software, formative, leading edge of what is happening. Coming along behind that is the hardware, the masculine engineering mentality.

This will continue until the leading edge outdistances the engineering mentality through breakthrough. This is what the shamanic hope is: that we can find a way to use chemicals in our bodies, use our voices, our thoughts, and our hands upon ourselves and each other; to transform ourselves without technology; to move into the realm of the imagination—on the natch as it were—with an interiorized psychopharmacologically applied technology that frees us in the imagination.

At the same time that this is going on the engineering mentality is going to set human societies in orbit around the earth/moon and the near planets. But there is a catch here for the engineering mentality which is that the very void that surrounds the planets exemplifies the enfolding, abyssal, feminine element. It is the mysterious Mama matrix of *Finnegan's Wake*. The mysterious Mama matrix is the universe, and there is no escaping that fact. But I think the engineering mentality, which will seek to change man into his machines, will have to be counterpoised by the psychedelic, earth-oriented, imagination-oriented side of consciousness, which will create then the potential for the spiritual marriage that will be the alchemical incubation of a new form of humanity; and this is not far away.

It can't be far away. It is a personal responsibility incumbent upon all of us to act to help create it. There is a definite obligation to examine the possibility of action, and to think clearly about self and other, language and world, past and future. For too long we have lived in a world defined by geography. If you are born in India, you will find out that the cosmos is one way. If you are born in Brooklyn, you find out it is something else. We need to transcend these localized grids of biological fate, which make us what we are but don't want to be. We can claim this higher level of freedom by the simple act of paying attention to being.

We must begin to send out ideological visions rather than be the consumers of them. We need to turn off the virtual internal televisions which are hooking us in to the tired cultural assumptions dictated from the Pentagon, Madison Avenue, and the corporate state. We need instead to turn on our modems and to begin to interact with like-minded people throughout the world and establish this new intellectual order which will be the salvation of the biosphere, I firmly believe. The Internet concretizes our collectivity, finally allowing people to feel the interrelatedness of their fates; feel that interrelatedness as a thing that transcends national divisions, ideological divisions. The net allows each of us to recover the experience of being part of the human family.

No reconstruction of society can be done without psychedelics because we have drifted so long without them. Surely we are the products of societies that have gone longer without psychedelics than any other culture in the world. It's been two thousand years since the Mystery was real at Eleusis and in that two thousand years we have wandered far, far into dysfunction and confusion. But we are the prodigal sons. We can redeem the ideal of shamanism from pre-technological social stasis and actually project it, perfect it, and travel with it out to the stars.

And if we don't, everything is lost. There is no standing still. There is only risk and commitment to these millennial aspirations and cultural goals, goals that have the potential to restore meaning and direction to our civilization. If this is not done we will fritter away our opportunity and be left prey to the destruction and the horrors of the typical future scenario.

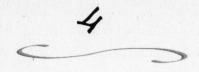

Two Classic Trips: Jean-Paul Sartre and Adelle Davis

Thomas Riedlinger

Although awareness of the use of hallucinogens by prominent individuals in society is generally restricted to the period of the counterculture of the late 1960s and early 1970s, these compounds were available earlier in the twentieth century. Jean-Paul Sartre, renowned French philosopher and a founder of Existentialism, had a single mescaline experience in 1935. He encountered a nightmarish vision, which clung to him for months after and became the inspiration for his acclaimed novel Nausea. *In this article, writer Thomas Riedlinger examines this poorly appreciated historical phenomenon. And, in contrast to Sartre's descent into psychochemical hell, Riedlinger also describes the exalted experiences of nutrition pioneer Adelle Davis in the late 1950s and early 1960s, catalyzed by LSD. From the terror of Sartre's* Nausea *to the religious epiphanies of Davis' "chemical Christianity," Riedlinger's description provides a glimpse into the profound impact these compounds have often had on influential figures of the last century.*

IN *THE MARRIAGE OF HEAVEN AND HELL*, William Blake wrote that the acids he used to etch poems and art work on printing plates were "salutary and medicinal, melting apparent surfaces away, and displaying the infinite which was hid." Modern users of a different kind of "acid," LSD, as well as other psychedelics, report a similar effect on human consciousness. These substances, they claim, can melt away the surface dross of daily life and manifest hidden dimensions of the spirit, or at least of the human unconscious.

Some find the experience positive, miraculous, a visionary rocket ride to heaven. For many, it's a terrifying plunge into the darkest depths of hell. Others experience both extremes, transcending the dichotomy by recognizing in it a dynamic union of sacred and profane. But one thing shared by most who brave the journey is a compelling urge to talk about it afterward. As Lester Grinspoon and James Bakalar note in their book *Psychedelic Drugs Reconsidered,* "it is as though words are never more necessary than when we approach the limits of language."

Not surprisingly, then, a review of recent catalogues from booksellers who specialize in drug-related literature discloses dozens of personal narratives describing the effects of psychedelics. Most of these works are mediocre; some are simply terrible. But scattered among them, like diamonds in clay, are a few undeniable classics of the genre, such as Aldous Huxley's *Doors of Perception,* Alan Watts' *Joyous Cosmology,* and Timothy Leary's *High Priest.*

On the other side of the coin, at least a few of the genre's classics aren't recognized as such. Among them are two representing, respectively, the hellish and heavenly potential of these substances. One is *Nausea,* Jean-Paul Sartre's 1938 existentialist novel that incorporates stark descriptions of the distorted perceptions and grueling emotions he suffered when he took mescaline in 1935. In his 1964 autobiography *The Words,* Sartre called himself "a chronicler of Hell" for having written it. The other work is *Exploring Inner Space* (1961), by "Jane Dunlap," a pseudonym for the nutritionist Adelle Davis, who took LSD five times in 1959 and 1960 in a quest for spiritual enlightenment, or, as she playfully put it, to get "chemical Christianity." The following looks at both books.

Nausea

Though still not widely recognized as such, Sartre's *Nausea* is unquestionably one of the greatest works of psychedelic literature. Insofar as it helped him win the 1964 Nobel Prize for Literature (which he refused), it is also the first truly world-class novel that reflects an author's personal experience with a hallucinogen other than cannabinols.

The mescaline experiment that so influenced *Nausea* took place in the early weeks of 1935. It was administered by injection in a hospital room in Le Havre, France, and resulted in a horrible experience. Sartre had asked his friend, the physician Daniel Lagache, to give him the drug to induce hallucinations so that he could explore his own consciousness. For several hours, Sartre thought himself under attack by giant octopuses, grinning apes, and huge, fat flies. An umbrella appeared to transform itself into a vulture, and a clock tower that he passed upon leaving the hospital seemed to turn into an owl. For months afterward, Sartre suffered flashbacks in which he imagined that he was pursued by giant lobsters. Though he realized that the lobsters were delusional, he feared he was losing his mind. It took almost a year for the lingering effects of his experiment with mescaline to disappear completely.

In "Sartre's Rite of Passage," my paper published in the *Journal of Transpersonal Psychology* in 1982, I traced a connection between the effects of Sartre's mescaline experiment and the content of *Nausea*, which he was writing at the time. This famous novel tells the story of a French academic named Roquentin who concludes that his life, and existence itself, are essentially meaningless. Though Sartre claimed in the late 1970s that what he described in the novel was not something he had actually experienced himself, he also stated in *The Words:* "At the age of thirty, I executed the masterstroke of writing in *Nausea*—quite sincerely, believe me—about the bitter unjustified existence of my fellowmen and of exonerating my own. I *was* Roquentin; I used him to show, without complacency, the texture of my life."

Roquentin's fictional life undoubtedly parallels Sartre's personal life in 1935. Like Sartre at the time, Roquentin is depicted as being a 30-year-old unpublished writer who's working on a book that represents the "only justification" for his existence. Also like Sartre, Roquentin is contemptuous of bourgeois society, feels himself getting older, and is starting to fear that his life will be wasted. The monotony of daily life oppresses him.

Early in the novel, Roquentin arranges a meeting with his former lover, Anny, whom he has not seen for several years. He hopes that the meeting will provide him with a *raison d'être* for his life. But before their reunion takes place, an event unfolds. It starts with what Roquentin calls "precursors of a new overthrow in my life." He is troubled by attacks of nausea (a common complaint during psychedelic sessions) and hallucinations that are vividly described in a number of colorful passages such as these:

There is a white hole in the wall, a mirror. It is a trap. I know I am going to be caught in it. . . . I draw my face closer until it touches the mirror. The eyes, nose and mouth disappear; nothing human is left. Brown wrinkles show on each side of the feverish swelled lips, crevices, mole holes. A silky white down covers the great slopes of the cheeks. . . . I plaster my left hand against my cheek, I pull the skin; I grimace at myself. An entire half of my face yields, the left half of the mouth twists and swells, uncovering a tooth, the eye opens on a white globe, on pink, bleeding flesh.

I was surrounded, seized by a slow, coloured mist, and a whirlpool of lights in the smoke, in the mirrors, in the booths glowing at the back of the café. . . . I was on the doorstep, I hesitated to go in and then there was a whirlpool, an eddy, a shadow passed across the ceiling and I felt myself pushed forward. I floated, dazed by the luminous fogs dragging me in all directions at once.

I see my hand spread out on the table. It lives—it is me. It opens, the fingers open and point. It is lying on its back. It shows me its fat belly. It looks like an animal turned upside down. The fingers are the paws. I amuse myself by moving them very rapidly, like the claws of a crab which has fallen on its back . . . I am my hand. I am these two beasts struggling at the end of my arms.

The crucial moment of the novel occurs when Roquentin wanders into a park and is distracted by a chestnut tree, its leaves and branches stirring in the wind. As he contemplates the tree's black roots that sink into the ground beneath the bench on which he's sitting, Roquentin cries out, "Suddenly, suddenly, the veil is torn away. I have understood, I have *seen*." What he has seen, in a transport of "horrible ecstasy," is that the tree is not what people call a tree. It exists in a pure state of Being outside of its name, its morphological characteristics, or the functions by which it is classified. As such it is essentially superfluous; the tree exists only to be.

In *The Doors of Perception,* Aldous Huxley reported a strikingly similar insight that occurred to him during his own, more pleasant mescaline experience. While gazing at some flowers that seemed to be shining with "their own inner light and all but quivering under the pressure of the significance with which they were charged," he concluded that what they "so intensely signified was nothing more, and nothing less, than what they were—a transience that was yet eternal life, a perpetual perishing that was at the same time pure Being."

For Roquentin, however, the existence represented by the chestnut tree has gravely different implications. If a thing has no reason for being except that it is, he reasons, its existence is not intensely significant, but absurd. Existence is a "universal burgeoning" of things that exist without reason, so existence itself is absurd:

Existence everywhere, infinitely, in excess, forever and everywhere; existence—which is limited only by existence. I sank down on the bench, stupefied, stunned by this profusion of beings without origin: everywhere blossomings, hatchings out, my ears buzzed with existence, my very flesh throbbed and opened, abandoned itself to this universal burgeoning. It was repugnant. But why, I thought, why so many existences, since they all looked alike? What good are so many duplicates of trees? So many existences missed, obstinately begun again and again missed—like the awkward efforts of an insect fallen on its back?

These questions are, of course, rhetorical. In the world according to Sartre, who professed to be an atheist since the age of ten, he and everything else that exists is superfluous; life had no ultimate purpose or meaning except what we choose to impose on it. Roquentin's existential crisis is to recognize this choice as artificial. In a vision that suddenly comes to him while he is sitting in the park, he perceives that the world is really a place of "soft, monstrous masses, all in disorder—naked, in a frightful, obscene nakedness," instead of being organized and solid as it appears to be.

Many people have experienced a similar upheaval on bad trips. Sartre's special genius was his ability to turn it into literature. The result is not only a novel about existentialism. *Nausea* also provides us with a picture of Sartre's psychological problems.

In an effort to better understand the source of these problems, my 1982 paper relied on a number of insights from Stanislav Grof's[1] psychedelic psychotherapy research and Sartre's description of his childhood in *The Words*. I tried to show that the texture and tone of the mescaline session revealed a lot about Sartre, in particular that he was haunted by excessive, morbid fears symptomatic of birth-trauma memories.

Such memories have been frequently reported by people who experienced "rebirthing" during Grof's psychedelic sessions, including many who said the phenomenon gave them "a fresh understanding and appreciation of existentialist philosophy" and especially the works of Sartre. Sartre himself dismissed birth-trauma theories as "highly fantastic." However, there seems little doubt that the pivotal park scene in *Nausea* concludes with a rebirth experience evoked by the mescaline:

Had I dreamed of this enormous presence? It was there, in the garden, toppled down into the trees, all soft, sticky, soiling everything, all thick, a jelly. And I was inside, I with the garden. I was frightened, furious, I thought it was so stupid, so out of place, I hated this ignoble mess. Mounting up, mounting up as high as the sky, spilling over, filling up everything with its gelatinous slither, and I could see depths and depths of it reaching far beyond the limits of the garden. . . . I was floating. I was not surprised, I knew it was the World, the naked World suddenly revealing itself, and I choked with rage at this gross, absurd being. . . . I shouted "filth! what rotten filth!" and shook myself to get rid of this sticky filth, but it held fast and there was so much, tons and tons of existence, endless: I stifled at the depths of this immense weariness. And then suddenly the park emptied as through a great hole . . .

Note the vivid descriptions of physical symptoms identified by Grof as being typical of the rebirthing phenomenon: a sensation of contact with biological material, such as blood, mucus, urine, and feces; rage and other violent emotions; severe breathing difficulties; a sense of entrapment; and the experience of passage through the birth canal into the world of light.

In the aftermath of this experience, Roquentin leaves the park and meets with Anny. She rebuffs his attempt to rekindle their old passion. "There is nothing more which attaches me to her," Roquentin says. Like Sartre's mother Anne-Marie in real life, Roquentin's lover Anny had "suddenly emptied herself" of him.

By the end of the novel, it's clear that Sartre blames his eponymous nausea on awareness of his own and other existences. Jack Kerouac, however, was perhaps a little closer to the truth in his famous novel *On the Road:*

The one thing that we yearn for in our living days, that makes us sigh and groan and undergo sweet nauseas of all kinds, is the remembrance of some lost bliss that we probably experienced in the womb and that can only be reproduced (though we hate to admit it) in death. But who wants to die?

Certainly not Sartre. That he was terrified of death throughout his childhood is openly admitted in *The Words,* where he reports being "frozen with fear" as a young boy when he read this account in a newspaper:

One summer evening, a sick woman, alone on the first floor of a
country house, is tossing about in bed. A chestnut tree pushes its
branches into the room through the open window. On the ground
floor, several persons are sitting and talking. . . . Suddenly someone
points to the chestnut tree: "Look at that! Can it be windy?" They are
surprised. They go out on the porch. Not a breath of air. Yet the
leaves are shaking. At that moment, a cry! The sick woman's husband
rushes upstairs and finds his wife sitting up in bed. She points to the
tree and falls over dead. The tree is as quiet as ever. What did she
see? A lunatic has escaped from the asylum. It must have been he,
hidden in the tree, who showed his grinning face. . . . And yet . . .
how is it that no one saw him go up or down? How is it that the dogs
didn't bark? . . . The writer starts a new paragraph and concludes, casually: "According to the people of the village, it was death that shook
the branches of the chestnut tree." I threw the paper aside, stamped
my foot, and cried aloud: "No! No!" My heart was bursting in my chest.

In *Nausea*, Sartre regurgitates this memory by casting the chestnut tree
of death in a central role. It represents what Susan Sontag, in *Against Interpretation*, calls "the fundamental problem of the assimilability of the
world in its repulsive, slimy, vacuous, or obtrusively substantial there-
ness—the problem that moves all of Sartre's writings." When Roquentin
concludes that the tree in the park is superfluous because it has no reason
to exist, the world around him dissolves into chaos; his consciousness finds
it impossibly hard to "assimilate" the concept of contingency and still
maintain a *Weltanschauung*. For Sartre, the tree's superfluity mirrors his
own. He believes that because we are doomed to eventually die, human
life is essentially meaningless; chaos lurks beneath our cozy but deluded
sense of meaningful involvement in the world. Sartre's mescaline experience exposed this hidden chaos and unleashed related fears of death and
madness, rejection and failure. Their manifestation in *Nausea* is entirely
consistent with Grof's psychedelic research and the findings of others who
have used these drugs in psychotherapeutic sessions. "Fear and anger bar
the way to the heavenly Other World and plunge the mescaline taker into

hell," observed Huxley in *Heaven and Hell.* Thus Sartre, though denied
paradisiacal pleasure, plunged into his personal hell and returned with a
book for the ages.

Exploring Inner Space

By the time of her death from bone cancer at age 70 on May 31, 1974,
Adelle Davis was to health food and nutrition what Rachel Carson is to environmentalism. She had been called a "supernutritionist" by *The New York
Times Magazine,* an "earth mother to the foodists" by *Life,* and a "spunky
preacher of the good-eating gospel" by *Time.* But her role as a writer of classic psychedelia is less well-known. *Who Was Who in America,* for example,
lists only her four books about nutrition and ignores the pseudonymous *Exploring Inner Space,* subtitled *Personal Experiences under LSD-25.*

This is probably no accident. Even today, so long after her death, Davis'
good reputation is a lucrative commodity. Her books on nutrition, most notably *Let's Eat Right to Keep Fit* (1954), have sold well over 10 million
copies and some remain in print. Her name still is used in promotional tie-
ins; a brand of seven-grain bread sold in grocery stores, for example, bears
a label proclaiming that it has been "made with a recipe by Adelle Davis."
That her estate seems disinclined to advertise the fact that she repeatedly
took LSD should therefore come as no surprise. When Cynthia Palmer
and Michael Horowitz asked permission to include a lengthy excerpt from
Exploring Inner Space in their landmark 1982 anthology *Shaman Woman,
Mainline Lady: Women's Writings on the Drug Experience,* their request
was summarily denied.[2]

No matter. Those who would silence this wonderful writer's psychedelic
voice can't put the toothpaste back in the tube. Her book is out there on library shelves and in secondhand bookstores, and is now and then listed in
the catalogues of rare-book dealers. When its copyright expires it will no
doubt be reprinted and enjoy a much wider readership. Until then it remains
a buried treasure for spiritual seekers, psychedelicists, and lovers of good
writing who are willing to invest some time and trouble in tracking it down.

For Davis, the chain of events leading up to her five LSD sessions

started in 1957, when she read about "magic mushrooms" in a *Life* magazine article written by R. Gordon Wasson, a vice-president at J.P. Morgan.
Wasson and his photographer Allan Richardson were the first "white out-
siders" invited to eat psilocybin mushrooms in a secret religious ceremony
held by Mazatec Indians living in a small, remote mountain village in Mexico. "As I read," recalled Davis, "I was overcome with an envy which refused to disappear."

The chance to do something about it came in 1959, when she approached the psychedelic psychotherapist Dr. Oscar Janiger and volunteered to take LSD in hope of "overcoming spiritual poverty" and to get
"chemical Christianity." She felt unfocused about her religious beliefs and
regretted to think she would never see God. Janiger and his associates
agreed to her request, with one stipulation: She had to record in detail her
visions while under the drug.

These visions unfolded according to general themes that were different
in each of the sessions. "The evolution of the soul" is how she characterized the first one. It took place on October 24, 1959, in the home of a psychiatrist who gave her 110 micrograms of LSD.

Initially, Davis listens to various musical recordings that evoke a wide
range of emotions, mainly sympathy for those who suffer loneliness. Then,
as the drug's effect deepens, she imagines herself changing form to become: every "terrorized, tortured human and beast" at the moment of
death; an amoeba in the ocean at the dawn of life on earth, dividing again
and again into millions of other single-celled creatures that evolve into life
forms of increasing complexity; and the first seed bursting open and growing, with great difficulty, upward through the rocky soil. Its tiny, green-
tipped shoot that breaches the surface symbolizes indomitable hope.

This plant proliferates, along with the protean animals, all of them enraptured by and reaching for the light of a distant sun that represents God.
The age of the dinosaurs arrives, and Davis finds herself becoming a variety of fearsome beasts "fighting in death struggles, consumed with hatred
and terror." They're attacking each other not mainly for food, but because
they're compelled by a fierce, primal cruelty.

Davis next changes into hundreds of volcanoes spewing lava that eradicates most life on earth, then "howling blizzards" and enormous, crushing glaciers. Her voice becomes "the sound of the wind . . . sobbing at such sheer desolation."

A luxuriant jungle appears, containing marshes in addition to huge trees and magnificent tropical flowers. Davis is now transformed into lions, gazelles, panthers, bright-plumed birds, and other animals in sequence. They still fight and kill, but for the purpose of survival rather than cruelty.

Suddenly, Davis runs out of the house and repeatedly vomits while lying on the grass of an adjoining garden. Later, after vomiting twice more, she concludes that the act is symbolic of humanity "trying to rid itself of the negative emotions" of primordial strife: "Because of man's ability thus to throw out negative feelings, from the snarling, hissing, and fighting, the catastrophes and the suffering, he had evolved to become capable of such positive emotions as forgiveness, compassion, kindness, mercy, honor, charity, self-sacrifice, and love."

With a great surge of joy, Davis grasps that all these positive emotions that exist in human beings are actually manifestations of God, and that her visions therefore represent "the very evolution of the soul." She comprehends that God, "Whom I had so long sought and, with the aid of LSD, had so quickly found, was the whole of this paradise which lay deep within each person."

For the second session two months later, Davis took a slightly stronger dose of LSD—150 micrograms. This time the dominant theme was "bejeweled fantasy," beginning with several visions reminiscent of scenes from the Disney film *Fantasia:* a female Pegasus flying through space, dancing snowflakes, a tiny fish with huge fins, fairies emerging as white-gowned seeds from milkweed pods in autumn, and a variety of musical instruments that generate abstract forms and colored light.

Davis then becomes a worried hen with her head near the ground, urgently searching for something beneath every leaf, and a mole rooting frantically underground. What are they looking for? she wonders. "God," both animals answer. "I burst into tears," Davis says, "feeling that I, like the hen and the mole, had spent my life looking for God in the wrong places and in the darkness."

Again as Pegasus, she sets out to find God. But the first thing she sees on her quest is an ancient Persian philosopher, the "composite of all scholars, professors, and philosophers of every age," who turns to stone before her eyes for having celebrated intellect too much while neglecting emotions. Feeling herself also starting to turn into stone, she soars back into space amidst millions of blazing stars that surround her in every direction. The universe is filled with celestial music. She revels in its perfect rhythm, galloping millions of light-years through space. Nowhere is darkness encountered. There is only "an endless sea of glorious golden light which was in truth God stretched into infinity," a light that both fills and surrounds all human beings. These "fantasies," Davis concludes,

> were like dreams in which one does not solve problems by rational thinking: yet a dream itself may be the solution to a problem. . . . At last I could see that when intellectual development is overemphasized, the subjective part of one's self, in which religious experiences occur, is usually undervalued; thus the finding of God is hindered by the worship of the intellect.

The third session, held on January 20, 1960, began with 150 micrograms of LSD. When Davis complained, untruthfully, that nothing appeared to be happening after an hour and a half, she was given an additional 50 micrograms that carried her mind into "whirlpool vortexes of ever-increasing magnitude, a terrifying experience even when richly rewarded."

This time the theme of her visions was "a cry for unseen beauty." After first becoming insects, such as a grasshopper, spider, and butterflies, then forests on mountains and plains, mighty rivers, streaks of lightning, and magnificent, roaring waterfalls, Davis is transformed into a silkworm representing all silkworms collectively. This marvelous creature also symbolizes her own hidden beauty and talents, spinning out "gigantic bolts of cloth thousands of yards wide, silks of exquisite colors such as surely no one has ever dreamed of." They cover the sky "from dome to horizon," swaying constantly as if in a gentle breeze and falling into graceful folds that catch the light and cast rich shadows.

The silkworm thus creates a wide variety of beauty in the world, such as sunrises, autumn colors, rainbows, and flowers. She tirelessly manufactures "snows which glistened in sunshine, woven with millions of diamonds; snows which sparkled in moonlight, sprinkled with star dust; blue snows which could be used for shadows, glaciers, and icebergs; and red, orange, yellow, and lavender snows which reflected the colors of sunrises, sunsets, and the aurora borealis." And there are mists of pastel light produced from cloth "inconceivably thin, soft, and silky," drifting gracefully to earth upon the mountain peaks.

In *Nausea,* Sartre asked sarcastically, "What good are so many duplicates of tree?" Davis here provides an answer when she says that as the silkworm, she was determined

> to dedicate all my energies to creating so much beauty that people would be forced to notice it. Just as fish must lay thousands of eggs so that one adult of their species might survive, or an oak must produce thousands of acorns so that a single tree might grow to maturity, I felt that I must create thousands of times more beauty than would ever be noticed. By doing so, I believed that at least a thousandth of this beauty would be appreciated.

Finally, after spinning massive quantities of cloth that represent all the human emotions, good and bad, the silkworm weaves a landscape that incorporates God's incorruptible golden light. Reverently gazing at the tall, golden mountains with burnished gold shadows and shimmering peaks, at the clouds of golden mist and spun gold rivers flowing tranquilly past golden trees and grainfields, Davis weeps at the realization that within her heart "love and beauty and God had become one."

In the fourth session, nineteen days later (February 8, 1960), on 150 micrograms of LSD, Davis finds herself transformed into a giant, luminous cobra that becomes at once her persona and her instructor. She starts in ancient India, observing the young Buddha in his father's royal garden, then travels through time and the world to see Jesus at the age of ten and Muhammad as a boy in Mecca. As she watches their various destinies unfold, she concludes that "the teachings of these three great religious leaders were amazingly similar" and that each embraced the same God.

Suddenly, the cobra orders Davis to confront buried feelings of fear that she'd rather avoid. It castigates her cowardice for failing to accept God's love and for seeking fulfillment instead in human love, material comforts, and her career. Each of these errors in turn is manifest symbolically as stoniness, coldness, and darkness.

"Accept your fear," counsels the cobra. "All persons are afraid. Everyone has wanted love thousands of times. Such wanting has brought disappointment and pain more often than not. The pain remains permanently recorded in your brain, and cumulatively it results in fear so great that being hurt again becomes intolerable."

After further expositions, Davis and the cobra return to ancient India and linger beneath the bodhi tree where the Buddha gained enlightenment. A "delicious harmony" there covers her "like a blanket, seeping into every pore." She senses that this harmony pervades the whole universe, hidden from us only by "our own warped feelings and our tragically myopic vision." But how can we quiet our fears enough to appreciate it? How can we learn to love selflessly?

The cobra answers with another vision. Davis finds herself standing with Christ in the Garden of Gethsemane. Also present, she notes, are discouragement, loneliness, sadness, and desolation. His crucifixion imminent, Christ prays that "if it be possible, let this cup pass from me." It is clear that he fears the ordeal ahead. Yet he rises and walks from the garden to accept his fate, teaching Davis that "Christ, by His death, had given each of us the courage to live."

The session concludes with a series of visions depicting Christ's sermons and miracles during his ministry. His exemplary tolerance, forgiveness, and humility give Davis additional courage. She finds that her previous deep-seated fears have been replaced by the conviction that she will never be alone, that God is with her always.

The fifth and final session took place fifteen days later, on February 23, 1960. Aware that her experiences so far had been visionary rather than classically mystical, Davis was determined to tap LSD's fullest potential for spiritual enrichment and prepared herself by reading the Bible, going to church, and meditating.

The dose again was 150 micrograms. In this session, Davis first becomes a speck of dust floating in a shaft of light in what appears to be the room in Mexico where Gordon Wasson ate the sacred mushrooms; then she is in churches and cathedrals all over the world. Soon, she says,

> I was floating in the silence of yet another shaft of sunlight, this time in a forest of giant redwoods. With eyes still filled with reverence and love, I could see God's strength in the dignity of the trees, God's glory in the blueness of the sky, and God's beauty in the lush greenness of the fern-covered ground. God's peace was in the whole, pervading alike trees, sky, ferns, and my soul, bringing both joy and sadness so great that tears could not be held back.

After other transformations, she becomes a drop of water "bubbling with carefree abandon in an underground spring" that emerges as a mountain stream. In winter she is trapped beneath an "opalescent layer of ice." In the spring, when it thaws, she's set free to rush "laughing, splashing, dancing, leaping, floating, eddying, and whirling through great canyons" en route to the sea, where she evaporates and falls to the earth as snowflakes and rain.

These visions, which Davis interprets as forms of "divine ecstasy," now move into the culminating mystical experience she's hoped for. Seeping underground, she finds that she is one of many water drops patiently lifting and dropping sharp stones, grains of sand, and bits of clay in the process of scooping out huge caverns that symbolize various aspects of the soul. She travels through them one by one and discovers humanity's untapped spiritual riches. Her vision includes a cave of dazzling gems that represents the hidden talents of all human beings. Another cave, containing a lake whose depths reflect a lapis lazuli and sapphire glow, represents the human collective unconscious with the answers to all of life's mysteries. Others, filled with phosphorescent stones and colored mists and alabaster, represent the sweetness and tenderness of God in every soul, the need for constant spiritual growth in addition to faith, the oneness that underlies all perceived opposites, and more such revelations.

This quick description belies both the grandeur of Davis's visions and the poignancy of her interpretations. There is no question that the caverns of the soul represent an apotheosis. They converge at the end of the session, transformed into pillars of luminous mist on a mountaintop. Below them is a burnished gold foundation; above, a golden roof. "The total appearance," Davis says, "was that of a sky-wide and sky-high acropolis, awesome in its magnitude. This I knew was the sacred temple of the soul, not of mine alone but of every human being who lives." At last she had come to the end of her journey and found that the spiritual edifice her intellect so often had attempted but failed to build already existed in her heart and in the depths of her soul.

After writing their two classic works, Sartre and Davis did not openly express a desire for further psychedelic explorations. An awkwardly translated line in *Sartre by Himself,* the published script of a film documentary, seems to indicate that Sartre tried mescaline again. But in a letter sent on March 13, 1984, I learned from his friend and lifelong companion Simone de Beauvoir that in fact it was a friend of his who later tried the drug and experienced pleasant hallucinations. Sartre himself, she wrote with emphasis, "*never* again took mescaline."

He did, however, gobble massive quantities of speed in the form of Corydrane, a European brand name for amphetamine, while working on his 1960 book *Critique of Dialectical Reason*. "I worked on it 10 hours a day, taking Corydrane," he reported in an interview published in *Life/Situations: Essays Written and Spoken.*

Near the end of the project, he said, he was taking twenty of the pills a day.

"I really felt that this book had to be finished," Sartre explained. "The amphetamines increased the speed of my thinking and writing so that it was at least three times my normal rhythm, and I wanted to go fast." His health suffered, but he used the drug again to write a three-volume study of the novelist Flaubert that was published in 1971–72. "I did an enormous amount of work, using Corydrane, on that book too," he recalled in the *Life/Situations* interview. "I spent 15 years on it, working on and off."

As for Davis, she said near the end of *Exploring Inner Space:* "If I had an Aladdin's lamp, I would make a wish that all persons who desired to take LSD could do so, and that I might be given it approximately twice each year." Later, in an article about her in *The New York Times Magazine* of May 20, 1973, a year before her death, she said she wouldn't take the drug again because she was concerned about reports, long since disproved, that it damaged human chromosomes. But she still called the LSD sessions described in her book a "marvelous, deeply religious experience."

Notes

1. From 1956 through 1973, Grof, a psychiatrist, personally conducted or participated in over 3500 psychotherapy sessions using LSD or other psychedelics, and reviewed the case histories of 1800 additional psychedelic sessions conducted by other researchers. His basic finding, first published in book form as *Realms of the Human Unconscious,* is that psychedelic drugs have a propensity to scan the unconscious like radar, lock onto areas of "high affective tension," and project the psychological content of those areas (e.g., memories of traumatic childhood incidents, including birth trauma) into consciousness.

2. Per Michael Horowitz. Personal communication with the author dated October 3, 1992.

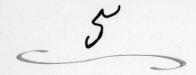

The Good Friday
Experiment

Huston Smith, Ph.D.

A fascinating event in the early history of hallucinogen research was The Good Friday Experiment. Conducted by Harvard psychiatrist Walter Pahnke, this study was designed to determine if hallucinogens could induce a genuine mystical experience. Administering psilocybin to ten divinity students and an inactive placebo to ten others, Pahnke demonstrated a powerful correlation between the active hallucinogen-induced state and the mystical experience. Huston Smith, one of Pahnke's subjects and at that time Professor of Comparative Religion at the Massachusetts Institute of Technology, describes in this recent interview with Thomas Roberts a little-known incident that occurred during the study, providing insight into the range of potential experience, positive and negative, induced by hallucinogens.

THOMAS ROBERTS

This is October First, 1996. Huston Smith will be telling us about an event that happened in the Good Friday Experiment in 1962. Huston, do you want to tell us about the student who ran out on the experiment?

HUSTON SMITH

Just keep me on course.

ROBERTS

O.K.

SMITH

The basic facts of the experiment have been recorded elsewhere and are fairly well known, but I will summarize them briefly. In the early sixties, Walter Pahnke, a medical doctor with strong interests in mysticism, wanted to augment his medical knowledge with a doctorate in religion. He had heard that the entheogens often occasion mystical experiences, so he decided to make that issue the subject of his research. He obtained the support of Howard Thurman, Dean of Marsh Chapel at Boston University, for his project, and also that of Walter Houston Clark who taught psychology of religion at Andover Newton Theological Seminary and shared Wally's interest in the entheogens.

Clark procured twenty volunteer subjects, mostly students from his seminary. Ten more volunteers, of whom I was one, were recruited as guides. Howard Thurman's two-and-a-half-hour 1962 Good Friday service at Boston University would be piped down to a small chapel in the basement of the building where the volunteers would participate in it. Fifteen of us would receive, double-blind, a dose of psilocybin, and the remaining fifteen a placebo: nicotinic acid, which produces a tingling sensation that could make its recipients think they had gotten the real thing. The day after the experiment we would write reports of our experiences, and Pahnke would have them scored by independent raters on a scale of from zero to three for the degree to which each subject's experience included the seven traits of mystical experience that W. T. Stace lists in his classic study, *Mysticism and Philosophy.* There was one borderline case, but apart from that, the experiences of those who received psilocybin were dramatically more mystical than those in the control group. I was one of those who received the psilocybin, and I will say a word about my experience before I proceed to the student that you asked about.

The experiment was powerful for me, and it left a permanent mark on my experienced worldview. (I say "experienced worldview" to distinguish it from what I think and believe the world is like.) For as long as I can remember I have believed in God, and I have experienced his presence both within the world and when the world was transcendentally eclipsed. But until the Good Friday Experiment, I had had no direct personal encounter with God of the sort that *bhakti yogis,* Pentecostals, and born-again Christians describe. The Good Friday Experiment changed that, presumably because the service focused on God as incarnate in Christ.

For me, the climax of the service came during a solo that was sung by a soprano whose voice (as it came to me through the prism of psilocybin) I can only describe as angelic. What she sang was no more than a simple hymn, but it entered my soul so deeply that its opening and closing verses have stayed with me ever since.

My times are in Thy hands, my God, I wish them there;
My life, my friends, my soul, I leave entirely in Thy care. . . .

My times are in Thy hands, I'll always trust in Thee;
And after death at Thy right hand I shall forever be.

In broad daylight those lines are not at all remarkable, but in the context of the experiment they said everything. The last three measures of each stanza ascended to a dominant seventh which the concluding tonic chord then resolved. This is as trite a way to end a melody as exists, but the context changed that totally. My mother was a music teacher, and she instilled in me an acute sensitivity to harmonic resonances. When that acquisition and my Christian nurturance converged on the Good Friday story under psilocybin, the gestalt transformed a routine musical progression into the most powerful cosmic homecoming I have ever experienced.

Having indicated how I experienced the service I can turn now to the incident that is the main point of this interview.

As the psilocybin began to take its effect, I became aware of a mounting disorder in the chapel. After all, half of our number were in a condition where social decorum meant nothing, and the other half were more interested in the spectacle that was unfolding before them than in the service proper. In any case, from out of this bizarre mix, one of our number emerged. He arose from his pew, walked up the aisle, and with uncertain steps mounted the chapel's modest pulpit. Thumbing through its Bible for a few moments, he proceeded to mumble a brief and incoherent homily, blessed the congregation with the sign of the cross, and started back to the rear entrance of the chapel and through its door.

Now, before the experiment began, we had been arranged in groups of four subjects plus two guides. We knew that two subjects and one guide in each group would receive psilocybin, and the guides were instructed to look after the others as needed. "John" (I withhold his actual name) was not my charge, but as no one got up to follow him, I did so.

This introduces an interesting parenthetical point. More than once I have been struck by the widely corroborated fact that however deep one may be into the chemical experience, short of the dissociation that John was experiencing, one can snap back to normal if need arises to so do. So it was in this case. When John's guide didn't respond to his leaving the chapel, I sprang to my feet and followed him out.

He had made a right turn and was striding down the hall, but that didn't worry me because we had been told that the entire basement had been sealed off for the experiment. But when he reached the door at the end of the corridor and jammed down its latch bar, it swung open. Something had misfired in the instructions to the janitor, and my charge, totally transported by his altered state, was loose on Commonwealth Avenue. I ran after him, but my remonstrances to return to the chapel fell on deaf ears, and he shook off my grip as if it were cobwebs.

What to do? I was afraid to leave him lest I lose track of him, but alone I was powerless to dissuade him from what appeared to be an appointed mission.

Providentially, help arrived from an unexpected quarter. Eva Pahnke, Wally's wife, was having a picnic on the grass with their child, and I shouted to her to keep track of John while I rushed back to the chapel for help. The strategy worked. When I returned on the double with Wally and another helper, John was still visible a block and a half ahead. Before we reached him we saw him enter what turned out to be 745 Commonwealth Avenue, the building that houses Boston University's School of Theology and parts of its College of Liberal Arts. We caught up with him on the stairs to the third floor, but Wally's remonstrances cut no more ice than mine had. Together, however, the three of us were able to block his further ascent.

Things were at a standstill when a postman rounded the corner of the steps from below. He was carrying a brown envelope copiously plastered with special-delivery stickers, and as he was passing us John's arm shot out and snatched it from him. I was too occupied to notice the expression on the postman's face, for two of us had all we could do pinning John's arms while finger by finger, Wally pried the crumpled envelope from John's vise-like grip and returned it to its stunned carrier. I have often wondered how that postman explained the mangled condition of his packet to its recipient, and how he described the incident to his wife at dinner that evening.

The rest is simply told. Realizing that he was overpowered—barely, for under the influence his strength was like Samson's—John, tightly flanked, submitted to being walked back to the chapel where Wally injected thorazine, an antidote. That returned him to his right mind, but with no recollection of what had happened. It took twenty-four hours for all the pieces of the episode to come back to him and fall into place, whereupon this was his story.

God, it emerged, had chosen him to announce to the world the dawning of the Messianic Age, a millennium of universal peace. (As often happens in such cases, the actual wording of the message made little sense to normal ears.) In his homily in the chapel, John broke the good news to our congregation, but he needed to get it to the world at large, which was what caused him to leave the chapel. When, walking down Commonwealth Avenue, he saw the plaque announcing "Dean of the College of Liberal Arts" by the entrance to 745 Commonwealth Avenue, it occurred to him that deans have influence, so if he could get to him, the dean would call a press conference that would complete John's mission. The postman's packet, he assumed, was for the dean, so if he attached himself to it, it would carry him to the dean himself.

John's long-term feelings about the experiment were heavily negative. He was the only one of its subjects who refused to participate in Rick Doblin's twenty-fifth-year retrospective study of the long-term effects of the experiment on its subjects, and he threatened to sue if his name was included.

ROBERTS

Was there something in Howard Thurman's sermon that prompted him to his messianic mission?

SMITH

Not to my notice. It was a typical Good Friday service with meditations on each of the seven last words of Christ. Howard Thurman was a remarkable man, both spiritually and in his ability to inspire people, but I don't remember the content of his words, only their moving impact. Did you ever meet him?

ROBERTS

No. I wish I had.

SMITH

Just relating this story I feel my spin tingling.

ROBERTS

Are there other memories of the afternoon that come to mind?

SMITH

I come back to the hubbub that erupted at times in our chapel. I was too deep into my own experience to be distracted by it, but I was peripherally aware of it and realized in retrospect that an observer would have found us a pretty unruly bunch. Half of us were enraptured, while the other half (as I learned from several of them the next day) felt left out and were not above acting out their resentment in derisive laughter and incredulous hoots over the way the rest of us were behaving.

I also recall a short exchange with one of our number in the foyer to the chapel just before the service began. I was already feeling my psilocybin, and sensing—wrongly, it turned out—that he was as well, I said to him from the depths of my being, "It's true, isn't it?" By "it," I meant the religious outlook, God and all that follows from God's reality. He didn't respond and told me when we next met that he had gotten only the placebo and hadn't a clue as to what I was talking about. So I was dead wrong in inferring from our eye contact that our minds were in sync.

ROBERTS

Anything else?

SMITH

Only the gratitude I feel toward Wally for having mounted the experiment—as you know, it's a poignant gratitude for he died nine years later in a tragic scuba diving accident. I have explained how it enlarged my understanding of God by affording me the only powerful experience I have had of his personal nature. I had known and firmly believed that God is love and that none of love's nuances could be absent from his infinite nature; but that God loves *me*, and I *him*, in the concrete way that human beings love individuals, each most wanting from the other what the other most wants to give and with everything that might distract from that holy relationship excluded from view—*that* relation with God I had never before had. It's the theistic mode that doesn't come naturally to me, but I have to say for it that its carryover topped those of my other entheogenic epiphanies. From somewhere between six weeks and three months (I should judge) I really *was* a better person—even at this remove, I remain confident of that. I slowed down a bit and was somewhat more considerate. I was able to some extent to prolong the realization that life really is a miracle, every moment of it, and that the only appropriate way to respond to the gift that we have been given is to be mindful of that gift at every moment and to be caring toward everyone we meet. To carry those sentiments with one onto the campus of the Massachusetts Institute of Technology requires empowerment.

ROBERTS

Thank you, Huston.

SMITH

You are welcome.

6

Chemical and Contemplative Ecstasy: Similarities and Differences

Roger Walsh, M.D., Ph.D.

Roger Walsh, professor of psychiatry, philosophy and anthropology at the University of California at Irvine and respected scholar on the phenomenology of religious experience, presents his views on the nature of the hallucinogen experience. Reviewing the long-standing debate over the validity of mystical experience induced by psychoactive drugs, Dr. Walsh reminds us that most societies possess institutionalized forms of altered states of consciousness, which among traditional peoples are almost always considered to be genuine spiritual experiences. Walsh proposes that it is the task of those having received personal illumination, regardless of mystical path, to return to the world so all may benefit from the light bestowed.

AFTER ALMOST A CENTURY of intellectual oblivion, consciousness has finally become a respectable topic for research. This does not mean that there is any agreement on what consciousness is. In fact, there is enor-

mous disagreement and controversy. However, most Western researchers—
be they philosophers, psychologists, or neuroscientists—subscribe to some
form of materialism, believing that consciousness is a product or aspect of
matter. Many contemplatives, on the other hand, hold a very different
view, usually some form of idealism, in which they believe that consciousness is the primary constituent of reality.

The fact that researchers and contemplatives hold very different views
about the nature of consciousness is not surprising since beliefs about the
nature of consciousness depend to a significant extent on one's range of experiences. Those people who have had transpersonal experiences tend to
be much more likely to view consciousness as a fundamental constituent
of reality. Small wonder then that two contemporary researchers, Hof-
stadter and Dennett, claimed "so far there is no good theory of consciousness. There is not even agreement about what a theory of consciousness
would be like. Some have gone so far as to deny that there is any real thing
for the term 'consciousness' to name."

Optimal States of Consciousness

Yet whatever consciousness is, the desire to alter one's experience or
state of it is clearly common. In a cross-cultural survey, the anthropologist
Erika Bourguignon found that 90 percent of the several hundred societies
she surveyed possessed institutionalized forms of altered states of consciousness. She concluded that this "represents a striking finding and suggests that we are, indeed, dealing with a matter of major importance, not
merely a list of anthropological esoterica." Moreover, she found that in traditional societies these altered states were viewed, almost without exception, as sacred. In his book *The Natural Mind*, Andrew Weil, one of the
leading researchers on psychoactive substances, concluded that the "desire to alter consciousness periodically is an innate normal drive analogous
to hunger or the sexual desire."

If human beings are innately driven to alter their consciousness, and if
fully 90 percent of societies have institutionalized altered states of consciousness, then this raises the obvious and important question of the na-

ture of the optimal state(s) of consciousness. This is the question I would like to discuss here, along with the related question of whether drugs can sometimes induce these optimal states.

In the West, it is commonly assumed that our usual waking state is optimal. Yet many contemplative traditions view consciousness as their central concern and make several claims that run counter to Western assumptions.

These include statements that:

1. Our usual state of consciousness is severely suboptimal;
2. Multiple states—including true "higher" states—exist;
3. These higher states are attained and stabilized through contemplative training.

Contemplatives claim unequivocally that our usual state of consciousness is not only suboptimal, it is dreamlike and illusory. They assert that we are prisoners of our own minds, unwittingly trapped by a continuous inner fantasy-dialogue which creates an all-consuming, illusory distortion of perception and reality. These traditions suggest that we live in a collective dream variously known as "maya," "illusion," or what the psychologist Charles Tart calls a "consensus trance."

Obviously, if these various philosophies and contemplative traditions regard our usual state as suboptimal, then they must regard some other state(s) as superior. Numerous traditions converge on the idea that the most valuable states are the classical mystical states of unitive consciousness. These include, for example, the yogi's samadhi, the Buddhist's nirvana, the Christian's union mystica, the Muslim's fana, and the Taoist's union with the Tao. In these states the usual egoic boundaries are transcended and the mystic feels at one with the universe.

Usually the state of mystical union is obtained after years or even decades of intensive practice of spiritual disciplines that center around mind-training. This mind-training aims to overcome the condition recognized by Sigmund Freud that "man is not even master in his own house . . . in his own mind." Of course, Freud was only echoing the lament of countless contemplatives who have made the same discovery. Some 2,000 years earlier Hinduism's *Bhagavad Gita* lamented:

> *Restless the mind is.*
> *So strongly shaken*
> *In the grip of the senses.*
> *Truly I think*
> *The wind is no wilder.*

This is why, as the great Hindu sage Ramana Maharshi said, "All scriptures without any exception proclaim that for attaining salvation mind should be subdued." For thousands of years, the royal road to the transpersonal was prolonged spiritual practice.

Chemical and Contemplative States

Yet with the advent of psychedelics in the West came a remarkable claim. Noncontemplatives who took these substances reported a vast range of experiences—some high, some low, some ecstatic, some demonic—but also some that seemed remarkably similar to those described by mystics across the centuries. This set off a debate which has raged ever since about the nature of this "chemical mysticism."

Proponents, such as the religious scholars Aldous Huxley, Walter Houston Clark, and Huston Smith, argued for the equivalence of chemical and natural mystical experiences. They based their argument on three things. First, on the experiential similarities between natural and chemical states; second, on the long use of psychedelics in various religions; and third, on experiments such as that of Walter Pahnke. In 1962, Pahnke administered psilocybin to theology students at the Harvard School of Divinity prior to a Good Friday church service. The experiences reported by the majority of the group given psilocybin were indistinguishable from reports of classical mystical experiences. Twenty-five years later, most of the psilocybin subjects "still considered their original experience to have had genuinely mystical elements and to have made a uniquely valuable contribution to their spiritual lives."

Others, including Arthur Koestler and the scholar of religions R. C. Zaehner disagreed. They argued vehemently against the possibility that a few milligrams or even micrograms of some chemical could possibly induce experiences that contemplatives labored decades to achieve. In his article "Do drugs have religious import?" which is the most frequently reprinted article in the history of *The American Journal of Philosophy,* Huston Smith considered the criticisms advanced against the equivalence of chemical and natural mysticism. His conclusion? These criticisms are unconvincing. The criticisms, and Smith's responses to them can be summarized as follows:

1. *Some drug experiences are clearly anything but mystical and beneficial.*

   Agreed! But this does not prove that *no* drug experiences are mystical and beneficial.

2. *The experiences induced by drugs are actually different from those of genuine mystics.*

   They are obviously different in causation, but, as the Harvard Good Friday study showed, they may be experientially indistinguishable.

3. *Mystical rapture is a gift of God that can never be brought under merely human control.*

   This argument, of course, is hardly likely to convince atheists, nontheists such as Buddhists, or Christians who believe more in the power of good works than of grace.

4. *Drug-induced experiences are too quick and easy to be considered identical to contemplatively induced experiences.*

   However, if the states are experientially indistinguishable, then the fact that they arise from different causes and with different degrees of ease may be irrelevant. The philosopher W. T. Stace has called this "the principle of causal indifference."

5. *The aftereffects of drug-induced experiences are different, less beneficial and less long-lasting than those of contemplatives.* Smith summarized this point eloquently, noting that while "drugs appear to

induce religious experiences, it is less evident that they can produce religious lives."

But the fact that aftereffects may be different does not necessarily mean that the experiences are.

Despite these arguments, the debate continues over whether drug-
induced mystical experiences are "really genuine." For example, the psychiatrist Stanislav Grof, who probably did more authorized clinical research
on psychedelics than anyone else wrote that "after thirty years of discussion, the question whether LSD and other psychedelics can induce genuine spiritual experiences is still open."

One reason why the debate continues is that there has been no adequate theory of mystical states that could resolve it. Let us then, first define mystical experiences, and then consider a theory that may help us
understand them.

For the purposes of this discussion, the term mystical experience will be
used to describe an altered state of consciousness characterized by:

1. Ineffability: the experience is of such power and so different from
   ordinary experience that it seems to at least partly defy description;
2. Heightened sense of understanding;
3. Altered perception of space and time;
4. Appreciation of the holistic, unitive integrated nature of the universe and one's unity with it;
5. Intense positive affect, sometimes including a sense of the per-
   fection of the universe.

Such experiences have been called by many names. In the West they
have been described, for example, as transpersonal experiences, as cosmic
consciousness by Richard Bucke, as peak experiences by Abraham Maslow,
as "numinous" experiences by Carl Jung, and as "holotropic" experiences by
Stan Grof. In the contemplative traditions, common terms include samadhi
(yoga), satori (zen), and fana (Sufism).

Tart's Model of Consciousness

What is needed is a theory accounting for the induction of similar states by such different means as LSD and meditation, followed by different aftereffects. It may now be possible to advance such a theory in light of current understanding of the induction of altered states of consciousness.

Charles Tart's model of consciousness is helpful here. Tart suggests that any state of consciousness is the result of the interaction of multiple psychological and neural processes such as perception, attention, emotions, and identity. If the functioning of any one process is changed sufficiently, the entire system or state of consciousness may shift.

It therefore seems possible that a specific altered state may be reached in more than one way by altering different processes. This reaching a common end point via different routes is an example of what general systems theorists call "equifinality." For example, states of calm may be reached by reducing muscle tension, visualizing restful scenery, or focusing attention on the breath. In each case, the brain-mind process used is different, while the resulting state is similar.

By analogy, it may be argued that a similar phenomenon could occur with mystical states. Different techniques might affect different brain-mind processes yet still result in the same, or at least very similar, mystical states of consciousness. For example, a contemplative might finally taste the bliss of mystical unity after years of cultivating qualities such as concentration, love, and compassion. Yet it is also possible that a psychedelic might affect chemical and neuronal processes so powerfully as to temporarily induce a similar state.

It seems that Tart's theory of consciousness may provide an explanation for the finding that "chemical mysticism" and natural mysticism may be experientially similar. But what of the fact that the long-term effects of the two may be different? These differences may also be compatible with the theory.

Both psychological and social factors may be involved. The psychedelic user may have a dramatic experience, perhaps the most dramatic of his or her entire life. But a single experience, no matter how powerful, may be insufficient to permanently overcome psychological habits conditioned over decades. The contemplative, on the other hand, may spend decades deliberately working to retrain habits along more spiritual lines. Thus when the breakthrough finally occurs, it visits a mind already prepared. In addition, the contemplative has acquired a belief system and worldview that explain the experience, a discipline that can cultivate it, a tradition and social group that support it, and an ethic to guide its expression. As Louis Pasteur observed, "chance favors the prepared mind." The contemplative's mind may be prepared, but there is no guarantee that the drug user's is.

This is not to say that the contemplative will always be transformed and the drug user never. Some psychedelic users may be psychologically and/ or spiritually mature and may be significantly transformed by their experience. Likewise some mystics may not be, or at least may have areas of personality, behavior and neuroses that remain relatively untransformed.

In summary, these ideas suggest that some drugs can indeed induce genuine mystical experiences in some people on some occasions. However, they are more likely to do so, and more likely to produce enduring benefits in prepared minds.

The Varieties of Mystical Experiences

Yet it may be that we can push our investigation a stage further. For it is becoming increasingly apparent that there is not just a single type, but rather multiple types, of mystical experiences. Careful mapping of mystical experiences may enable us to identify states which are in reality quite different, yet have not been distinguished in the past. For example, the states induced by yoga, shamanism, and Buddhist meditation have sometimes been described as identical. Yet careful comparison of the experiences shows that they may be quite distinct.

The general principle seems to be that different contemplative techniques are more likely to induce certain types of mystical experiences than others. For example, zoom shamans may experience a sense of unity with the world (nature mysticism), whereas Theravadin Buddhist meditators aim for an experience of nirvana in which all objects and phenomena of any kind disappear and only consciousness remains. Careful studies may show that specific psychedelics are more likely to facilitate certain mystical states than others. Perhaps we will find that the more advanced the state, the less likely it is to occur, whether spontaneously, contemplatively, or chemically. LSD and analogous substances, for example, may induce experiences of nature mysticism more often than nirvanic experiences.

In addition, different classes of psychoactive substances will likely induce different classes of states. For example, empathogens such as MDMA (Adam, ecstasy), which are reputed to have strong emotional effects and may induce feelings of love, may be more likely to foster corresponding mystical experiences. Clearly a further level of sensitivity and discernment may be possible in research on mystical experiences, however they are induced.

States and Stages: Stabilizing Mystical Experiences

For those people who are graced with a mystical experience—whether spontaneous, contemplative, or chemical—the crucial question is what to do with it. It can be allowed to fade, be ignored, or even dismissed, or perhaps clung to as a psychological/spiritual trophy. On the other hand, it can be consciously used as a source of inspiration and guidance to direct one's life along more beneficial and beneficent directions.

One such direction, indeed the direction recommended by the great mystics, is to undertake the necessary contemplative training of life and mind so as to be able to reenter and extend the mystical state. The aim is to extend a single peak experience to a recurring plateau experience, to stabilize a state of consciousness into a stage of development, to change an altered state into an altered trait, or as Huston Smith put it so eloquently, to transform flashes of illumination into abiding light.

The method for this stabilization is spiritual practice. Authentic spiritual disciplines—ones capable of producing transpersonal development—are essential for stabilizing deep insights and transformations. Without them there is little chance that deep experiences will fulfill their remarkable potential for psychological and spiritual health, well-being, maturation, and contribution to others.

Authentic spiritual disciplines contain at best seven central practices and produce seven corresponding benefits. These practices are 1) redirecting motivation away from mundane obsessions to self-transcending goals; 2) transforming emotions, by weakening destructive emotions such as fear, anger, jealousy, and strengthening beneficial ones such as love, joy, and compassion; 3) living ethically; 4) fostering concentration; 5) refining awareness; 6) cultivating wisdom; and 7) developing generosity and altruism. These constitute the seven central and essential "perennial practices" at the heart of the great religions.

Even the experience of abiding light is not the endpoint of the journey. For beyond personal realizations—whether it be called enlightenment, liberation, satori, salvation, Ruach Hakodesh, moksha, or fana—lies the stage of sharing that realization with the world. The wisdom and illumination that have been gained are now used to teach, serve, help and heal. The mythologist Joseph Campbell described this as "the hero's return," and there are numerous descriptions of it in the world's religious traditions. In Zen, it is called "entering the marketplace with help bestowing hands" and in Christianity, as "the fruitfulness of the soul" According to the Hindu sage Ramakrishna, people at this stage:

> are constantly engaged, inwardly or outwardly, in the humble service
> of all creatures, whom they experience as transparent and beautiful
> vessels of the one Presence. In their holy company, the longing to
> know and merge with Truth arises and intensifies naturally.

In summary, our challenge is to open to the experience of illumination, however it occurs, then to stabilize that illumination through contemplative practice, and to bring its light back to the world for the benefit of all.

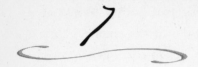

Drugs and Jewish Spirituality

That Was Then, This is Now

Lawrence Bush

Lawrence Bush, a writer and editor of Jewish literature and art, describes the not uncommon experience of those who experimented with hallucinogens in the sixties and encountered a profound challenge to their rational world view. Writing three decades later from his experiences as a young seeker, Bush reflects on how the hallucinogens may be integrated into Jewish theology and mysticism. Bush critiques current drug education policies, and concludes that "Just Say No" propaganda ultimately interferes with parents' rights to guide and protect their children. In this sensitive article, Bush shares his insights on how the challenge of the hallucinogen experience may be resolved through faith.

1.

Rabbi Kahana explained an inconsistency: the word for "wine" is spelled tirash but pronounced tirosh. If a man merits it, wine makes him rosh, "chief"; if not, it makes him rash, "a poor man."

Rava explained another inconsistency: as spelled, the text reads, "Wine that desolates [yeshammah]" (Ps. 104:15), *but we pronounce the last word, "yesammah* [that maketh glad]." *If a man merits it, wine makes him glad; if not, it desolates him. That is what Rava meant when he said: Wine and spices stimulate my mind.*

—Babylonian Talmud, Yoma 76b,
in H.N. Bialkik & Y.H. Ravnitzky, *Sefer Ha-Aggadah*

The first time I ever stayed up all night and saw daylight return, I was seventeen years old and "tripping" on LSD. The solidity of the New York cityscape as dawn spread through the streets was profoundly comforting to me: after the radical shifts in perception that I had weathered through the night, here I could affirm that the world does not dissolve during the hours of sleep, but "remains the same forever" (Eccles. 1:4).

Uncertainty about such existential fundamentals eventually drove me to abandon LSD and all other drugs. By dint of personal wiring and family history, I was lacking in *emunah,* the faith to know that I could have such experiences and land in a grounded reality. Looking back, today, on the twenty-plus "acid trips" that I took as a much-too-young adult, I sort them into two varieties. At their most gentle, psychedelic drugs evoked some superb sensory experiences: the half-hour examination of the exquisite symmetry of a dew-hung spiderweb, the glimpsing of a smile on a trotting dog's face, the sudden apprehension of cubism as a form of realism. "Hallucination" belittles these experiences: dogs, after all, *do* smile.

More problematic were the "mystical" moments, tinged with madness, that involved a greatly intensified sense of metaphor and meaning, the dissolution of ego borders, the powerful "perception" of what was real and illusory, natural and bizarre, holy and profane—and the manic longing to organize these insights into a redemptive system. Such episodes, deeply challenging to the rationalism that my family held dear, would leave me incapacitated by ambivalence. *Bouncing ego can't be free, boundless ego won't be me,* I wrote in a poem at age eighteen. And so, like the Hebrew people at the foot of Sinai, I "fell back and stood at a distance" ("Let not God speak to us, lest we die," Exod. 20:15–16). I left psychedelic drugs behind, far less with a sense of relief than with a sense of failure, incompleteness, and envy for those free spirits who *could* safely ascend the mountain.

Such Jewish imagery probably would not have occurred to me during my drug-using days, when I identified more with the Woodstock Nation than with the Jewish People. Today, however, I do know more than one rabbi and Jewish professional who either postponed or extended the baby-boomer rite of drug experimentation to a time when Jewish metaphors came naturally to them. Their psychedelic experiences thus became tightly interwoven with their Judaism and deeply influenced their professional practice.

Rabbi C., for example, never took LSD during the sixties heyday, but waited until he was in his late forties. With his own rabbi serving as his (drug-free) "guide," C. spent some six hours rapturously experiencing the Revelation at Sinai. He had an overpowering sense of *devekut,* oceanic union with God; he could "see" the entire cosmos, micro and macro, and experienced what he calls "an unbearable feeling" of having his own boundaries stretched to encompass it all. This piercing perception of the infinitesimal yet infinite nature of his individual identity was accompanied by an overpowering infusion of faith, a certainty about there being meaning in the universe and interconnection among all life. This mystical encounter served as the bedrock of Rabbi C.'s creative theology for the next eighteen years. "What I experienced and felt," he reports, "was not unreal or less real but *more* real than my daily perception of reality. I've never felt any other way about it."

Another rabbi, N., an executive within Jewish organizational life, was a weekly user of marijuana and hashish and "tripped" several times annually for a twelve-year period before entering rabbinic school. Rabbi N. believes that "drug experiences opened me up for prayer experiences and a relationship to God—there are even similar feelings of community in getting high with people and praying with them." He especially deplores the criminalization of drugs in America, which has made drug use into "the leading source of crime and waste of government money." Instead, N. believes, "a way should be found to allow marijuana and psychedelics to expand people's spiritual consciousness in a safe environment."

A Jewish educator and day school principal, B. took psychedelic drugs about a dozen times, "always with a sense of spiritual mission." She remembers a Shavuot some twenty years ago when she and three other women (all prominent in Jewish life today) "borrowed" a Torah scroll from a day school ("It was locked away on Shavuot!"), took it to a state park, ate hallucinogenic mushrooms and spent the day reading Torah, along with "woodland creatures, frogs, and deer," who "came out and participated!" B. admits that "the fact of connectedness or 'oneness' that the *Sh'ma* expresses first became clear to me on LSD."

A successful editor of Jewish books, F. had numerous psychedelic experiences in the 1970s. "I look back on nearly all of them with great awe and respect," F. says. "Each time was a 'big occasion' with a consistent teaching: that there are all kinds of things going on in the spectrum that my normal waking consciousness doesn't pick up. It's like a dog whistle—your ear doesn't hear all frequencies. But with each 'awakening' there is some residue left in the senses, as with the lightning bolt described by Rambam [Maimonides], which briefly illuminates the sky."

A third rabbi, J., who heads a vibrant congregation in the Northeast, undertook two LSD experiences during and shortly after college and feels that they strongly influenced his later rabbinic practice. "I remember sitting outside our apartment in the snow," reports J., "drawing a circle in the snow to make a pie, putting jelly on it, cutting up slices and eating them. Looking through the patio doors of the next apartment, I saw a very fancy cocktail party. I realized at that moment that every social interaction is a construct, a kind of pretense. The perception didn't require me to 'drop out,' but it did help make me radically unregimented as a rabbi. I saw that there is no particular activity or time that has a meaning beyond that which we humans have attached to it. Nothing is sacred, in other words, except when we choose to make it sacred—which is something I really value and love doing."

2.

Were the great ritual moments of Judaism used as reminders (or recreators) of states of elevated consciousness, as they once were used to some extent by the Kabbalists, those of us who have gained religious insight through the use of drugs might indeed find great excitement in the ritual life.

—Rabbi Arthur Green, writing pseudonymously
as Itzik Lodzer, in *Response,* Winter 1968

The Jews I have quoted are certainly among the more radical in contemporary Jewish life. They are hardly alone among baby-boomer Jews, however, in their experiments with psychedelic drugs and their positive associations between those experiments and their Jewish spirituality. Nor are such Jews limited to the liberal denominations: "I know many *ba'alei teshuvah,*" reports F., speaking of Orthodox and Hasidic friends and neighbors, "who cannot deny that their spiritual journey included 'getting high with a little help from their friends.'"

"Awakenings" via drugs have often led to a desire to awaken Judaism itself. In particular, many psychedelic voyagers have spent subsequent years pushing against what Rabbi Arthur Green called, in his thirty-year-old *Response* article, the "cult of God-as-father" that "has been allowed to run rampant for hundreds of years" in Jewish life. "As presented today," wrote Green,

Judaism . . . has lost the creative mystic drive which led beyond its own images into a confrontation with the Nothing *[Ein Sof]*. The Judaism which contemporary Jews have inherited is one of a father figure who looms so large that one dare not *try* to look beyond Him. We have indeed become trapped by our image.

This trap, according to Rabbi Green, guaranteed that "most psychedelic voyagers" in the 1960s, including Jews, "sought their religious guidance in the traditions of the East," which encourage altered states of consciousness and are tolerant of fluid images of divinity. Against such a backdrop, the creative metaphysics of tripping (what Green called "the construction of elaborate and often beautiful systems of imagery which momentarily seem to contain all the meaning of life") seemed less heretical and more resonant.

Green's article proceeded to offer an alternative to the stodgy ol' Judaism of the 1960s by drawing four analogies between psychedelic drugs and kabbalistic mysticism. First, he wrote, the "everything-has-been-changing-but-nothing-has-changed" experience of tripping is analogous to "the Kabbalists' descriptions of God as *Sefirot*," in which "there is no limit to the ever-flowing and ever-changing face of the divine personality." Second, LSD's "terribly exhilarating liberation . . . from the bondage of all those daily ego problems" has analogy in Judaism's "'stripping off of the physical' (*Hitpashtut ha-Gashmiyut*)," an "interpretation that some of the Kabbalists give to the act of fasting on Yom Kippur." Third, the acid-induced sense of time as a "union of moment and eternity" is parallel to the kabbalistic view that "all future moments were contained within creation, and creation is renewed in every moment."

Finally, Green wrote of "the deepest, simplest, and most radical insight of psychedelic/mystic consciousness . . . the realization that all reality is one with the Divine." Despite Judaism's built-in "fears and reservations" about this insight, he declared, "the feeling of the true oneness of God and man is encountered with surprising frequency in the literature of the Kabbalah."

This theology of immanence (God is everywhere) is a typical hallmark of many Jews whose résumés have "LSD" invisibly written in the white space between the lines. So is a deep interest in Jewish mysticism and a desire to broaden the Jewish agenda from survivalism/group solidarity to "God-consciousness" and spiritually meaningful observance. To the extent that these interests have become pervasive among a wide variety of Jews, so do we glimpse their influence.

Yet the impact of psychedelic drugs on these innovators goes unacknowledged, even three decades after Rabbi Green's ground-breaking article. Perhaps his analogy between drugs and Jewish mysticism holds here, too, as the Talmud (Hagiga 13a) warns that "The things that are as sweet as honey," i.e., arcane knowledge, "should remain under your tongue." Most tongues have been tied less by reverence, however, than by the "Just Say No" propaganda of the past two decades, which has made saying "yes" or even "maybe" into a major career risk. It seems you cannot become president—not even in the Conference of Presidents of Major American Jewish Organizations—if you admit to having inhaled.

3.

Our masters taught: Four men entered the Garden, namely, Ben Azzai, Ben Zoma, Aher, and Rabbi Akiva. . . . Ben Azzai cast a look and died. . . . Ben Zoma looked and became demented. . . . Aher mutilated the shoots. Rabbi Akiva departed unhurt.

—Babylonian Talmud, Hagaig, 14b
in H.N. Bialkik & Y.H. Ravnitsky,
Sefer Ha-Aggadah/The Book of Legends

There is no stronger antidote to the intoxication of youth than the fears accompanying parenthood, and when I contemplate the prospect of my children (twelve-year-old boy/girl twins) "entering the Garden," I become very sober.

The hazards are many. An LSD trip is not an amusement park ride, delivering safe thrills within set parameters; it is an intense, day-long experience of altered brain chemistry, and its outcomes are strongly influenced by many factors, both subjective and environmental. Psychosis and exaltation walk side by side; the dissolving of ego borders and the uprooting from mental certainties can be terrifying, even lethal. The thirteenth-century Jewish kabbalist Abraham Abulafia could easily have been discussing LSD when he wrote of "spirits of jealousy" that gathered around him during his own mystical "trip," even as "God touched my mouth" and "a spirit of holiness fluttered through me." Over the course of the next fifteen years, "I was confronted with fantasy and error," Abulafia admitted. "My mind was totally confused, since I could not find anyone else like me, who would teach me the correct path. I was therefore like a blind man, groping around at noon" and "Satan was at my right hand to mislead me" (Tr. by Aryeh Kaplan; see Diane M. Sharon's essay in *The Fifty-Eighth Century,* ed. by Shohama Wiener, 1996).

Beyond psychosis, I dread having my kids physically injured or even killed while intoxicated by misjudging their own physical limits, disregarding the laws of physics, or simply driving a car. Although LSD is known for its peculiar virtue of provoking fantastic visions while maintaining an objective, "watcher" frame of mind, I would not want my children's lives to depend on the steadfastness of that "watcher." Instead, *I* want to serve as their watcher: the principle of *s'yag l'Torah,* making a fence around the Torah, has no greater application for me than in protecting the lives of my children through prudent parenting.

It is, however, the criminalization of drugs, rather than their inherent dangers, that most prevents me from serving as "watcher" over my children's safety and mental health. Certainly, the hostile policies of America have kept me from discussing drug use in as honest and nuanced a way as I would like with my kids, for fear that their naïve interpretations and adolescent gossip might lead to serious stigmatization, despite our being a drug-free household. As a result, their main source of drug education has been their school's DARE program (Drug Abuse Resistance Education)— a program awash with a repressive mystique that violates my values, while its deterrence power is very questionable. My own father, a pharmacist with detailed knowledge about the dangers of drugs, gave up a two-pack-a-day cigarette habit in the 1960s to deter my drug use by example. If such intimate heroism failed to halt my experimentation, why should a local sheriff's corny propaganda be effective?

Criminalization further assures that if my kids ever do mess with drugs, I will be helpless to assure "quality control" and maximize their safety. They will be left to procure their substances from whatever unsavory sources, in whatever dosages, for use in whatever environments, because they will lack my cooperation and guidance—guidance that could lead me to prison and loss of custody. American law thus throws up a huge wall between me and my children and all but assures that the spiritual possibilities of their drug use, if it transpires, will be seriously compromised.

What about Jewish law? "I brought the issue of substance use to a teacher of mine in the traditional world," reports F., the editor. "He told me there are two problems. The small problem is that the *halachah* teaches us to be lawabiding: *dina malkhuta dina,* 'the law of the land is the law.' The larger problem is embodied in the question: Who is the master and who is the servant?"

F.'s rebbe was talking about addiction—a scourge that directly challenges my open-mindedness about drug use. Drug and alcohol addiction, after all, are powerful catalysts of crime and social blight. Statistics on child abuse, domestic violence, rape, robbery, and murder reveal the central role addiction plays in facilitating human misery.

Advocates for the legalization of "soft" drugs, moreover, strike me as naïve when they deny that there is any link between use of marijuana and psychedelics and use of the harder stuff. "Sin begins as a spider's web and becomes a ship's rope," teaches Rabbi Akiva in *Genesis Rabbah* (22.6). Even as a reasonably sensible, self-aware, and middle-class pothead in the sixties, I tried almost every available drug at least once, including cocaine, amphetamines, tranquilizers, opium, and angel dust (nasty!). Only heroin, with its reputation for addictiveness, fatal overdose, and nausea for novices, provoked me to "Just Say No."

Addiction is not limited, moreover, to "hard" drugs. Several of my friends, for example, became psychologically "addicted" to marijuana well into their mature years. The narcissistic qualities of getting high—the sense of achievement, loosened inhibition, personal brilliance and hilarity—provided a buffer against the frustrations of thwarted ambition, relational *ennui,* and existential boredom that most human beings face. Only when these individuals realized that a plunge into the depths of humility was prerequisite to their growth were they able to stop medicating themselves.

Is their drug use fundamentally different or somehow less reprehensible than those of inner-city folk who smoke crack to rise above their blighted landscapes? The truth is that any drug, whether used to "awaken" the soul or to "deaden" it (a very subjective and culturally determined distinction), can be overused and misused. And all such abuse, to my mind, deserves a compassionate, psycho-spiritual response. Criminalization simply maximizes the degradation of the human beings involved—and turns my parental fears into nightmares.

4.

When I can undergo the deepest cosmic experience via some miniscule quantity of organic alkaloids or LSD, then the whole validity of my ontological assertions is in doubt. [Yet the] psychedelic experience can be not only a challenge but a support of my faith. After seeing what really happens at the point where all is One . . . I can also see Judaism in a new and amazing light. The questions to which the Torah is the answer are recovered in me.

—Rabbi Zalman M. Schachter,
writing in a *Commentary* symposium
on "The State of Jewish Belief," August 1966

Apart from legal impediments, why shouldn't psychedelic drugs be used in Jewish life as they have been in other faith traditions—as a tool for wrenching open the mind and heart to "God's presence"? Why not embrace the spiritual power of the psychedelic experience and try to elevate it, as we do with sexuality, above the recreational and into the sacramental zone? Why shouldn't the roster to Jewish life-passages include the opportunity to have a psychedelic experience (perhaps after the age of forty, Judaism's traditional age of enlightenment and mystical initiation, or perhaps at an earlier stage of development)—with rabbinic guidance and community approval? If Abraham's Voice and Moses' Burning Bush and the Revelation at Sinai are the archetypal encounters that inform our faith, why not strive to recreate such experiences throughout our "nation of priests"?

One "why not" is rooted in a spiritual work ethic. Arthur Green put it as follows in a second article in *Response,* published three years after his pseudonymous one: "That which you don't work out on your own, in a struggle that has to begin way down here in the world of ordinary weekday consciousness, somehow just isn't going to last."

True, LSD is promiscuous in its power: you needn't read Hebrew, study Torah, or make any Jewish commitments before you stand on "holy ground." The logic of banning such a powerful tool of religious awakening, however, would also have us banning English translations of holy texts, cross-referenced CD-ROM versions of the Talmud, and all such tools of "easy" access—as well as outreach strategies that seek to provide Jewish contexts for people's "real life" passions and hobbies (Jewish elder hostels, Jewish environmentalism, Jewish ski weekends, etc.). Jewish life has simply moved too far in the direction of democratization and cross-cultural pollination to retreat now.

Another "why not" targets mysticism itself. Writing in *Contemporary Jewish Religious Thought* (ed. by Arthur A. Cohen and Paul Mendes-Flohr, 1987), the late Israeli philosopher Yeshayahu Leibowitz devoted his entire essay on "Idolatry" to a denunciation of mysticism, which "is another name for idolatry." In particular, he wrote, the kabbalistic *sephirot,* which are "thoroughly imbued with . . . aspects of the divine . . . directly contradicts the scriptural view of God," which ascribes holiness to God and to nothing else. "How difficult it is," Leibowitz continued,

> for man *[sic]* to accept the distinction between the holy and the profane, between the creator, who alone is "truly real" . . . and utterly holy, and his own status in God's world, which is contingent and profane.

Such a critique, though rare in contemporary Judaism, has dogged Jewish mysticism for centuries. In particular, the Hasidic flowering of the mid-1700s was violently opposed by traditionalists (the *Mitnaggedim*) who viewed the Hasidic emphasis on ecstatic worship over study and *mitzvot* as heretical and idolatrous. Similarly, Rabbi C.'s LSD-induced experience of *devekut,* B.'s conviction that "connectedness and oneness" is the meaning of the *Sh'ma,* and Rabbi J.'s humanistic perception that "nothing is sacred, except when we choose to make it sacred," would all likely have been denounced by the Gaon of Vilna, leader of the *Mitnaggedim*—or by Yeshayahu Leibowitz—as egotism writ large.

Mysticism nevertheless seems integral to the spiritual upsurge of the 1990s. For better or worse, "getting high on God" far outweighs "submitting to the yoke of the *mitzvot*" in most Jewish circles, while courses in Kabbalah, meditation, and other Jewish techniques of consciousness expansion have full enrollments. Unless our community turns away, *en masse,* from this quest to "get high" through Jewish ritual, there is little ground here for excluding psychedelic explorations from our sacramental roster.

The fact is that psychedelic drugs have already been part of the "sacramental roster" for many baby-boomer Jews, who sensed while under the influence that "Surely the Lord is present in this place, and I did not know it!" (Gen. 28:16). Rather than emulating Jacob and erecting a pillar at the site of their discovery, they have been forced by two decades of repressive social policy to bury and hide it. Like the Marranos of old, they have bought respectability and influence with silence—a choice that has facilitated many innovations in American Jewish life. But that silence has also left our children to fend for themselves. It has left psychedelic voyagers without a Jewish port-of-call—and tens of thousands of human beings to wallow in prison without Jewish protest. It has left the heritage of the sixties vulnerable to slander, while the "War on Drugs" rages out of control, with inquisitors and cowards calling the shots.

"Truth is the center of the circle," wrote Abraham Ibn Ezra, the world-wandering Hebrew poet, commentator, and holy man of the twelfth century. Perhaps the time has come to step into Ibn Ezra's circle, face outwards to America, and admit to having inhaled.

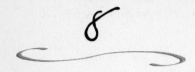

Using
Psychedelics
Wisely

Myron J. Stolaroff

In this article, Myron Stolaroff reviews the structures and considerations necessary to optimize safety during the hallucinogen experience. Stolaroff, whose experience with hallucinogens dates back to his collaboration with Willis Harman's study of the effects of LSD and mescaline on creativity, shares some of the insights he has acquired over four decades of personal experience. Examining concerns such as set and setting, motivation, intention and ethical integrity, Stolaroff is quick to point out that this path is not for everyone. Working through deep, repressed unconscious material, the Shadow of Jungian psychology, hallucinogens may overwhelm the psychic defenses of poorly prepared individuals and catalyze severe anxiety states. Emphasizing the value of integrating hallucinogen work into a disciplined spiritual path, Stolaroff presents a framework that he believes will minimize risks while optimizing beneficial outcome.

MY WIFE JEAN AND I had driven several miles up the mountain to an elevation of 6000 feet a few miles south of Mount Whitney in California.

We were about to meet Franklin Merrell-Wolff, author of the book *Pathways through to Space,* an impressively articulate and detailed description of a person entering a state of enlightenment and savoring it over several months.

When we were ushered into his private office, we found ourselves before an outstanding personage who radiated a marvelous glow. When we had talked for a few minutes and I felt sufficiently at home, I spoke of our research work, telling him that we had spent three and a half years administering LSD, sometimes in conjunction with mescaline, to 350 research subjects and had published our findings in medical journals.

"My oh my!" he said, looking at us with consternation. "I hope you haven't used these drugs yourselves."

We admitted that we had. He continued, "According to X" (here he mentioned an Indian sage whose name I do not remember), "it will take you seven incarnations to recover from the damage of taking such substances!"

Naturally I was upset, but I didn't think of the appropriate reply until we were driving back down the hill: "Never underestimate the grace of God!"

There is no question that psychedelic substances are remarkable graces. The farther one can reach into the vastness to be explored, the more one realizes how powerful these materials are. There seems to be no end to the levels of awareness that can be realized by those who use them to explore their psyches with integrity and courage.

The great value in these chemicals is that, in some way still not scientifically explained, they dissolve the boundaries to the unconscious mind. They give us access to our repressed and forgotten material, to the Shadow that C. G. Jung so effectively dealt with, to the archetypes of humanity, to an enormous range of levels of thought, and to the wellspring of creativity and mystical experience that Jung called the collective unconscious.

At the heart of the unconscious is what many experience as the source of life itself, and which some call God. Those who have experienced this describe it as a wondrous, ineffable source of light and energy that infuses all of creation, embracing all wisdom and radiating a vast, unending, and ever-constant love. Immersion in this is the essence of the mystical experience and produces what the great mystics have described as the state of unity or oneness. Such union is the culmination of all seeking, all desire; it is the most cherished of all experiences of which man is capable.

Not all who ingest these substances can count on such revelations. In fact, psychedelics are powerful agents and can be misused. It must be remembered that they help reveal the unconscious, and most of us have made its contents unconscious for very specific reasons. We may not welcome the appearance of repressed, painful feelings, or of evidence that our values and lifestyles might be considerably improved. Nor is it always easy to accept the spaciousness of our being, our immense potential, and the responsibility that these entail. We may also refuse to believe that we are entitled to so much beauty and joy without paying any price other than being ourselves!

To assure a rewarding outcome, let's look at some factors that should be taken into consideration when using these materials. I must add here that in no way am I encouraging the use of illegal substances. I do hope, however, that greater understanding of these materials will help restore an intelligent policy that will make further research possible. Here are some things that will help ensure beneficial results:

Set and Setting

Set and setting have been widely recognized as the two most important factors in undertaking a psychedelic experience. Of these, set has the greatest influence.

As the drug opens the door to the unconscious, huge spectrums of possibilities of experience present themselves. Just how one steers through this vast maze depends mostly upon set. Set includes the contents of the personal unconscious, which is essentially the record of all one's life experience. It also includes one's walls of conditioning, which determine the freedom with which one can move through various vistas. Another important aspect of set consists of one's values, attitudes, and aspirations. These will influence the direction of attention and determine how one will deal with the psychic material encountered.

In fact, one can learn a great deal by accepting and reconciling oneself with uncomfortable material. Resisting this discomfort, on the other hand, can greatly intensify the level of pain, leading to disturbing, unsatisfactory experiences, or even psychotic attempts at escape. This latter dynamic is largely responsible for the medical profession's view of these materials as psychotomimetic. On the other hand, surrender, acceptance, gratitude, and appreciation can result in continual opening, expansion, and fulfillment.

Setting, or the environment in which the experience takes place, can also greatly influence the experience, since subjects are often very suggestible under psychedelics. Inspiring ritual, a beautiful natural setting, stimulating artwork, and interesting objects to examine can focus one's attention on rewarding areas. Most important of all is an experienced, compassionate guide who is very familiar with the process. His mere presence establishes a stable energy field that helps the subject remain centered. The guide can be very helpful should the subject get stuck in uncomfortable places, and can ask intelligent questions that will help resolve difficulties, as well as suggesting fruitful directions of exploration that the subject might have otherwise overlooked. The user will also find that simply sharing what is happening with an understanding listener will produce greater clarity and comfort. Finally, a good companion knows that the best guide is one's own inner being, which should not be interfered with unless help is genuinely needed and sought.

Motivation

This is extremely important. Those who earnestly seek knowledge and deeply appreciate life in all its forms will do well. Yet certain characteristics of psychedelics make them very popular for recreational use. The most attractive of these is their great enhancement of sensual responses, which offer heightened perception, amplification of beauty and meaning, and intensified sensual gratification. Psychedelics can also generate a great sense of closeness among participants, especially in a group setting. While I am convinced that one of the great cosmic commands is "Enjoy," there are traps in using these substances purely for recreation. The first is that a person seeking the delights of the senses may find himself overwhelmed by the eruption of repressed unconscious material without knowing how to deal with it. Another danger is that constant pleasure-seeking without giving anything back to life can distort the personality and ultimately produce more discomfort. The safe, sure way to rewarding outcomes with psychedelics is through intelligent, well-informed use.

Honesty

For the serious spiritual seeker, or for that matter anyone seeking knowledge, the single most important characteristic is honesty. This means the courage to look at whatever is presented by the deep mind, the ability to admit one's shortcomings when they become apparent, and the determination to change one's behavior in line with the truth one has experienced.

Ongoing Discipline

Experts in the field now generally agree that it is wise to conduct psychedelic explorations within the framework of a spiritual discipline or growth program that will continually call attention to fundamental values and goals. A good discipline will outline a body of ethics for personal behavior that will support the changes required. Good ethics will also help us stay clear about our objectives, and will keep the door open to increasing depths of experience. Moreover, there is evidence to suggest that the more we are prepared to pass on to others whatever spiritual largess we have accumulated, the more we will be given.

For myself, I found training in Tibetan Buddhist meditation a potent adjunct to psychedelic exploration. In learning to hold my mind empty, I became aware that other levels of reality would more readily manifest. It was only in absolute stillness, accompanied by a special, highly developed quality of listening, that many subtle but extremely valuable nuances of reality appeared. While I achieved this to some extent in ordinary practice, I found this effect to be greatly amplified while under the influence of a psychedelic substance. This in turn intensified my daily meditation practice.

Psychedelics as Way-Showers

The role of psychedelics is often misunderstood. Many feel that having had wonderful experiences, they now have the answers and are somehow changed. And no doubt in many respects they are. But users often overlook the fact that there are usually heavy walls of conditioning and ignorance separating the surface mind from the core of our being. It is a blessing that psychedelics can set aside these barriers and give access to our real Self. But unless one is committed to the changes indicated, old habits of personality can rapidly reestablish themselves.

At this point many feel that repeating the experience will maintain the exalted state. It may, but most often real change requires hard work and dedicated effort. Unfortunately this is not always clear during the experience itself; it has merely pointed the way and shown what is possible. If we like what we see, it is now up to us to bring about the changes indicated.

There is a grace period following profound psychedelic experiences when changes can be rapidly made. At this time one is infused with the wonder and power of the new information. Moreover—and this is an area where some valuable research can be done—the drug experience releases a great deal of bodily and psychic armoring that is tied to our neuroses. This rejuvenation is quite noticeable after a good psychedelic experience, when, without the dragging weight of physical habit patterns, behavior can be more readily changed.

On the other hand, if you make no effort to change, old habits rapidly reassert themselves, and you find yourself sliding back into your previous state. In fact, it can be worse than before, because now you know that things can be better and are disappointed to find yourself mucking around in the same old garbage.

Another factor makes this process even more uncomfortable. A lot of the energy formerly tied up in repressed material is now released. This energy may be used quite fruitfully to expand the boundaries of your being to the new dimensions you have experienced. But if you return to old patterns of behavior, you now have more energy to reinforce them, making life more difficult. For this reason, these experiences must not be taken lightly, but with serious intent.

Dealing with the Shadow

As Jung indicated, the Shadow holds all the material that we have pushed aside so we can hide from ourselves. Unfortunately, it also contains much of our energy, and as long as it is unconscious, it exerts a powerful influence on our behavior without our knowing it. Furthermore, Shadow material is responsible for most of the difficulties humans create in the world. We project our Shadow onto others, believe those others to be the source of our difficulties, and seek refuge from them rather than taking responsibility in our own hands. Consequently we must resolve Shadow material if we are to develop. If this were accomplished on a widespread basis, it would be a major benefit for the world.

Jung describes human development as the process of "making the unconscious conscious." Psychedelics, particularly in low doses, can be an extremely effective tool in this process. The bulk of my experience is with the phenethylamine compounds, which remained legal longer than the standard psychedelics such as LSD, mescaline, and psilocybin. Whereas a full dose of a phenethylamine like 2C-T-2 or 2C-T-7 might be 20 milligrams, a low dose would be ten or twelve milligrams, or roughly equivalent to 25–50 micrograms of LSD.

The most infallible guide to Shadow material is our uncomfortable feelings. Many do not like to use low doses because these feelings come to the surface. Rather than experience them, they use larger doses to transcend them. But these uncomfortable feelings are precisely what we must resolve to free ourselves from the Shadow, gain strength and energy, and function more comfortably and competently in the world. By using smaller amounts and being willing to focus our full attention on whatever feelings arise and breathe through them, we find that these feelings eventually dissolve, often with fresh insight and understanding of our personal dynamics. The release of such material permits an expansion of awareness and energy. If we work persistently to clear away repressed areas, we can enter the same sublime states that are available with larger doses—with an important additional gain. Having resolved our uncomfortable feelings, we are in a much better position to maintain a high state of clarity and functioning in day-to-day life.

I would also like to add a word about frequency: Individuals vary greatly in their frequency of use of these materials. Some are satisfied with an overwhelming experience which they feel is good for a lifetime. Others wish to renew their acquaintance with these areas once or twice a year. Still others are interested in frequent explorations to continually push their knowledge forward. Regardless of the frequency, it is wise to make sure that the previous experience has been well integrated before embarking on the next one. Early in one's contact with these substances, where there is a wealth of new experience, this may take several months. As one becomes more experienced, the integration time grows shorter, and the interval between trials may be shortened.

Many stop the use of psychedelics when they feel they have learned what they wished. But often it is likely that they halt because they have hit a deeply repressed, painful area that is heavily defended. The issue goes beyond purely personal material, however. One is unlikely to reach full realization without awareness, not merely of one's own pain and suffering, but of that of all mankind. This may help explain the Dark Night of the Soul, which is the final barrier to mystical union described by Evelyn Underhill in her classic book *Mysticism*. Since we are one, we must not only confront the personal Shadow, but the Shadow of all humanity. We can do this more readily when we discover the ample love that is available to dissolve all Shadow material.

Freeing Constricted Areas

There is another way in which psychedelics can serve the serious seeker. It often happens that those pursuing rigorous spiritual disciplines achieve elevated states by pushing aside or walling off certain aspects of behavior. With honest use, psychedelics will not permit such areas to remain hidden, but will insist upon their surfacing. One then experiences the great relief of being in touch with all aspects of one's being. The joy and thrill of being totally alive come from having complete access to all of one's feelings.

The Trained User

There appears to be a cosmic law that says that giving our complete attention to an object, image, or idea with constancy, patience, and acceptance will allow its different attributes to unfold. Psychedelics greatly accelerate this process. To operate most effectively, the observer must have developed the ability to hold his mind steady so he can watch the process develop. Large doses can push one so hard that it is most difficult to do this. Therefore the best results are achieved by a "trained user"—a person who has learned to manage a high dose of psychedelics, or who has learned to hold his mind steady enough to observe his inner process competently. As a user clears up his "inner stuff," he gains more freedom in directing his experience. At this stage, higher doses can be profitably used to penetrate deeper into the nature of Reality.

Interestingly, this concept of the trained user does not appear in the literature. But it is precisely the trained user who can best take advantage of the unfathomed range of wisdom and understanding contained in the far reaches of the mind. There seems to be no limit to the dimensions of understanding that can be experienced by the explorer who has the courage, integrity, and skill to navigate them. With integrity, and with the support of appropriate disciplines and friends, one can bring back a great deal for the betterment of oneself and mankind.

Are psychedelics necessary? Can't these same explorations be conducted by those who have mastered the skills of meditation? No doubt they can—with an enormous investment of time and effort. But it is unlikely that many Westerners will be willing to make such a commitment. For Western seekers, whose spiritual practice must usually be integrated with making a living, the proper use of psychedelics can considerably accelerate the process. However, it is not a path for everyone. Choice should be based on full knowledge of the factors involved.

Psychedelics are not a shortcut, as it is of little value to sidetrack important experiences. If enlightenment requires resolution of unconscious material (and my personal experience indicates that it does), those who aspire to such achievement must carefully consider the pace and intensity with which they are willing to encounter this vast range of dynamics. The psychedelic path, while much more intense than many other disciplines, is in a sense easier because it often provides an earlier and more profound contact with the numinous. Such contact inspires commitment and opens the door to more grace in surmounting uncomfortable material.

If our commitment is truly to the well-being and happiness of all sentient beings, then it is reasonable to study all useful tools for accomplishing these ends. Psychedelics, used with good motivation, skill, and integrity, can contribute much toward easing the pain and suffering of the world while giving access to wisdom and compassion for spiritual development.

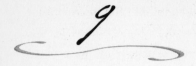

Successful Outcome of a Single LSD Treatment in a Chronically Dysfunctional Man

Gary Fisher, Ph.D.

During the 1950s and 1960s, hallucinogens were utilized in a variety of treatment settings, often for conditions which were nonresponsive to conventional therapies. An active investigator during this period was Gary Fisher, a psychologist at the UCLA School of Medicine. Dr. Fisher, describing his clinical work during this period administering hallucinogens to a variety of patient populations, including individuals with terminal cancer and children with infantile autism, has provided lucid accounts of this treatment modality. In this provocative paper, Fisher illustrates how hallucinogens may catalyze a therapeutic response, even in cases where it is least expected.

IN THE 1960s I was conducting an LSD research project at a West Coast medical center on the use of LSD for intractable pain in terminally ill cancer patients.[1] During this project the head of the Department of Psychiatry asked me if I thought it possible to "work in" an LSD treatment for the son of a CEO of a major corporation in the city. The message I got was to be cooperative. I met with the father and he told me that his son had had extensive and prolonged psychiatric treatment. He had been hospitalized at two of the country's most prestigious private psychiatric institutions but after eleven years of hospitalization and intensive psychoanalytic work no changes had occurred. For the following four years he saw a number of psychiatrists, tried every psychiatric drug available and even had a series of electro-shock treatments. The only procedure that he had not endured was psycho-surgery and the father was most reluctant to think about that alternative. The son was twenty-nine years old at the time, and had been in the psychiatric world for over fifteen years. He had never finished high school, never had a job and never had any friends. He had numerous diagnoses from a host of diagnosticians ranging from chronic schizophrenia to severe narcissistic character disorder. He never improved from any treatments, currently was not in treatment, and had run out of options. Although he had had numerous medications currently he was not being medicated because they made him feel worse. There was never any history of illegal drug usage. He spent his day in a darkened room constantly accompanied by a male psychiatric nurse. His activities were restricted to listening to the radio, watching TV, some reading, playing cards, and eating. The father requested that I see him at their home as the son refused to leave the house.

When I saw David he was almost friendly but a little aloof and formal. He had obviously read extensively in the psychiatric literature, and named off multiple symptoms from which he was suffering. His presenting symptoms included being phobic about most things in the world, in a constant state of anxiety and fear, unable to sleep (having night terrors if he slept) and experiencing a constant range of distressing bodily sensations and recurring feelings of loss of reality. On interview, although he was loquacious, his affect was shallow and his self-descriptions were rehearsed—he was an old hand at being interviewed by psychotherapists. He was pleased at having attention again as after his two prolonged hospitalizations he had been secluded for two to three years in his room with his attendant, not even venturing to other parts of the house or yard. He did not evidence signs of acute psychosis. He elaborated in great detail about all the prestigious people and institutions where he had been treated, always ending with a sad and heavy resignation that they hadn't been able to help him. He had no memory deficit and could describe in detail the variety of professional people that he had encountered. After about two hours he queried me as to my credentials—my academic vita, experience, training and professional affiliations. He obviously didn't want to be treated by a nobody, only collecting trophies of victory worthy of him. Evidently I met his standards as he said he would cooperate with the LSD treatment. After my meeting with him I assessed him as "the most untreatable psychiatric patient in the world." His father was an enormously successful, famous and powerful person, but David was, too. He would go down in history as the man who defied the psychiatric world to treat him. This was his claim to fame. The contest read David vs. LSD and, I wondered, who would win this one?

Preparation

My attempts at conducting our standard pre-session preparation were to no avail as he showed no interest in hearing about how this work was done. The session room was set up with the standard regime of music, flowers, artwork, artifacts from nature and tasty food morsels. Two other experienced sitters attended the session. The session was conducted in private quarters in a closed psychiatric ward of a large urban hospital. The format of the session was that developed by Hubbard[2] and the Saskatchewan group[3] with the key concepts of "set and setting," the focus of the endeavor being that the individual experience a transcendental state of consciousness. Sherwood, Stolaroff and Harmon precisely describe this process:

The concept underlying this approach is that an individual can have a single experience which is so profound and impressive that his life experiences in the months and years that follow become a continuing growth process . . .

There appears to emerge a universal central perception, apparently inde-
pendent of subjects' previous philosophical or theological inclinations, which
plays a dominant role in the healing process. This central perception, appar-
ently of all who penetrate deeply in their explorations, is that behind the ap-
parent multiplicity of things in the world of science and common sense there
is a single reality, in speaking of which it seems appropriate to use such words
as infinite and eternal. All beings are seen to be united in this Being . . .

Much of the "psychotherapeutic" changes are seen to occur as a process of
the following kind of experience:

The individual's conviction that he is, in essence, an imperishable self
rather than a destructible ego, brings about the most profound reorientation at
the deeper levels of personality. He perceives illimitable worth in this essential
self, and it becomes easier to accept the previously known self as an imper-
fect reflection of this. The many conflicts which are rooted in lack of self-
acceptance are cut off at the source, and the associated neurotic behavior
patterns die away. (p. 77)[4]

The Session Begins

Since he was so resistant to change, I felt he needed full dosage: 600
micrograms of LSD.[5] I suggested he lie down, relax, close his eyes and go
with the music. He declined this offer saying that he preferred to sit up but
after a few moments, observing that the sitters were going to close their
eyes and listen to the music and not engage him in small talk, out of boredom he picked up one of the art books and began casually leafing through
it. I had told him the session would last many hours, at least eight and possibly up to twelve, so he knew he had a lot of time to kill.

After about thirty minutes he began to look stressed. He was obviously
feeling the effects of the drug and I asked him what he was beginning to
experience, explaining that it would be helpful to communicate the changes
he was experiencing so that I could give him some hints about how to use
these changes. He pulled himself together and quickly said "Nothing's
happening." And that was that. So it went. He squirmed, trembled,
sweated profusely, his eyes bugged out, he turned blotchy red, hyperventi-

lated and looked like he was going to explode. To any of my gentle queries he responded with a firm "Nothing's happening." Finally he said, "Since nothing's happening I think I will just lie down for a while and listen to the music." The other two sitters and I simultaneously chorused, "Good idea." He lay on the couch; clenching his jaws and his fists, he would shake, perspire, groan, moan, make feeble guttural noises and then jolt back into the present time, look over at me and in a weak, feeble voice, say "Nothing's happening." This was turning out to be one of the most heart-wrenching LSD sessions I had ever sat through. We knew there was nothing we could do but wait for him. We waited ten hours and his position never shifted. For the complete time, he never appeared to have any respite from this intense agony. He was totally exhausted and looked absolutely devastated. After ten hours, all he could mutter was, "I guess this drug doesn't work with some people" and all I could manage was, "Well, we don't know a lot about this treatment yet. We all have a lot to learn." Both sitters and I agreed we had seldom experienced such an exhausting session. He stayed in the hospital overnight with his private attendant.

"Nothing Happened"

I met with him the next morning and he appeared overwhelmed with fatigue, still maintaining that he had no reaction whatsoever to the drug. During this follow-up meeting, I casually mentioned that because of all the different medications he had taken over the years, perhaps he had become drug intolerant and needed a second session with a much higher dosage. At this news he went stark white and was totally speechless. I then said that this one treatment was a special circumstance set up just for him and that we were not able to do further work with him in this hospital. That information got him breathing again and he looked as though he had just received reprieve from a death sentence. I mentioned that a colleague of mine had a private hospital in Holland where he used LSD and other psychedelic compounds in a series of treatments over a number of months. I suggested that he consider this if I was able to make such arrangements with this psychiatrist. Visibly shaken by this proposal he finally muttered that his father would probably not consider financially supporting such a costly undertaking, especially since he had absolutely no response to his first treatment. I left it at that, indicating I would contact my Dutch friend [Dr. G.W. Arendsen-Hein] to see if he could accommodate him if his father was amenable to the expense.

My Dutch colleague agreed to treat this man at his residential hospital near Ederveen, Holland, with the stipulation that I accompany him and participate in the first three sessions. I agreed and next contacted David's father who agreed to finance the venture.* I called David and told him that I had been successful in arranging this treatment program for him. He said he could not fly alone, that I would have to accompany him. I explained that had already been arranged and I would stay in Holland for his first three sessions. After a very long silence David agreed but said he could not go until he had attended to a number of personal matters. I asked him to let me know when he thought he would be ready to leave. That telephone conversation was the last contact I ever had with him.

In about three days I called his house and his mother answered. David was out and she was most anxious to talk to me. She said he had gone out by himself the day after my conversation with him—this was the first time he had gone out in several years. He had told her that when I called to tell me that he would call me when he was prepared to set a date to leave, as he was busy attending to personal matters. He did not inform her as to the nature of these personal matters, but she was so ecstatic that he was going out of the house that she didn't want to "push it." I called in about a week, also not wanting to push it. She answered again and reported that he was gone a good part of every day but when he was home he told her that if I called to tell me that he was resting but that he would call me back. He was always either out or resting when I called.

---

*An interesting aside that baffled both David and his father was that I never charged for any of my services. I felt that this fact was an additional phenomenon that helped penetrate David's view of the psychiatric world wherein therapists' only interest in him was for his monetary value. He never raised the issue, nor did I.

David Moves Out

After a couple of months of this he moved out of his parents' home to his own apartment and started to do volunteer work in a library. His mother contacted me, updating me on his new life and his father called me on two occasions, saying that one LSD treatment had produced more results than the previous fifteen years of psychotherapy. To his parents, LSD was a miracle drug. After about a year I stopped contact with David's mother. At that time he had a part-time job, still did volunteer work at the library and she was sure that he had a girlfriend but he wasn't very communicative about his activities. He made contact with them on his terms and limited to the times he set. They didn't push him. My understanding of some of this was pretty simple. He couldn't tolerate another LSD session; whatever he went through he knew he couldn't do that again. He also couldn't lose face and he was fortunate in having parents who were so grateful for the changes that had occurred that they didn't require explanations from him about what had happened.

Since David chose not to divulge his experiences, one can only hypothesize what occurred. Clearly he had been in great turmoil and severe anguish throughout his session. Observationally he had what is popularly referred to as "a bad trip." A bad trip is when an individual uses all his energies into combating the pending loss of ego control. The ego, in fighting to stay identified with what is "known," creates a living hell—everything turns to negations, everything is experienced as threatening and dangerous. All of the rejected aspects of the self are projected onto the external world and one experiences "reality" as demonic—such is the stuff of psychosis.* David undoubtedly had endless duels with his devils. The central

---

*Common experience among seasoned psychedelic voyagers in that the nitty-gritty psychodynamic work is accomplished during so-called "bad trips": that is, where the condition of one's humanity is illuminated. Having pleasant aesthetic and sensory experiences is important for people who never experience such phenomena, but for the usual person, a pleasant ego time doesn't touch the hidden internal conflicts which cause the difficulties in life.

and challenging question remains: "Why did David decide to change his life, to give up his "uniqueness" in the world and join the human condition with the rest of us?" His circumstances allowed him to remain at home living his life as he had lived it—being uniquely "untreatable" and that LSD therapy would be just another unsuccessful attempt to change him.

I posit that he saw what a horrific price he was paying to maintain this ego position; he saw his "victory" as empty; that his special place in the world was a meaningless one. That he took on the task of going out into the world he had left as an early teenager is quite astounding; that he did it on his own, even more astounding. It was a testament to the strength of his ego. Part of his unwillingness to share with me the results of his treatment session could have been that he identified me as a father. I was a powerful person who had powerful "medicine" and powerful connections. He wasn't quite ready to embrace as an ally this kind of potency—he was more willing to take on the world at his pace and on his own terms. I suspect that he knew that I knew something about this world of altered consciousness, that I was dedicated to help him explore it, and this was a mystery to him but he was not ready to take on this task. He decided he would rather become an "ordinary" person.

From the first day I met David I never treated him as a "patient," I never engaged him at the level that he had always functioned—therapist and patient. I treated him as though he were a perfectly rational and sane person. I never talked "therapy talk" with him, never interpreted any of his behavior, never psychoanalyzed him. I was always respectful of him, never played the role of the doctor, and although I listened to whatever he said I never responded or engaged in any conversation related to his psychopathology. I was very quiet with him and any comments I did make were extremely benign.

Although almost nothing is known of this man's experiences with the nonordinary realities induced by the drug, what we do know is that profound changes occurred in his behavior following these experiences; he became a functional human being after fifteen years of extreme dysfunctional behavior—this was a remarkable phenomenon.

Addendum

The purpose in reporting this case study has been to give testimony to the fact that psychedelics are powerful tools for an individual to use in accessing those forces in his psyche which determine the course of his life. In the revelations that occur in these states of expanded consciousness, one had the opportunity to explore and understand what is needed to be known in order to acknowledge the essential worth of the self and to discover the humanistic-spiritual existential "laws."

These processes are the same for everyone, regardless of one's status in life's many hierarchies. One's station or condition in life is not at issue—only at issue is the proper use of these materials administered in a safe and protected environment by sitters who have traveled the path of self-discovery themselves and know that each person can, with the help of enlightened guidance, achieve profound depth of understanding.

References

1. Fisher, G. Psychotherapy for the dying: principles and illustrations with special reference to the utilization of LSD. *Omega,* 1970, 1, 3–16.

2. MacLean, J.R., MacDonald, P.C., Byrne, V.P. and Hybbard, A.M. The use of LSD-25 in the Treatment of Alcoholism and other Psychiatric Problems. *Quart. J. of Studies of Alcoholism,* 1961, 22, 34–45.

3. Blewett, D.B. and Chwelos, N. *Handbook for the Therapeutic Use of LSD-25: Individual and Group Procedures.* Unpublished Manuscript; Regina, Saskatchewan, 1959.

4. Sherwood, J.N., Stolaroff, M.J. and Harmon, W.W. The Psychedelic Experience—A New Concept in Psychotherapy. *Journal of Neuropsychiatry,* 1962, 4, 69–80.

5. Fisher, G. Some comments concerning dosage levels of psychedelic compounds for psychotherapeutic experiences. *The Psychedelic Review,* 1963, 1, 208–218.

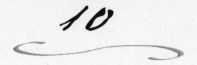

Sitting for Sessions: Dharma & DMT Research

Rick J. Strassman, M.D.

Rick Strassman was the first psychiatrist in twenty years to receive permission in the 1990s to research hallucinogens. While at the University of New Mexico School of Medicine, Dr. Strassman investigated the physiological and psychological effects of the powerful synthetic hallucinogen, dimethyltryptamine (DMT), administered intravenously. In this account, Strassman examines and integrates the range of responses his subjects experienced within the Buddhist perspective. A long-standing Zen practitioner, Strassman also presents the conflictual relationship the American Buddhist community has had with hallucinogen research, and his views on how these tensions may be resolved.

IT IS JANUARY 1991, twenty-three minutes after I injected a large dose of DMT (N,N-dimethyltryptamine) into Elena's arm vein. Elena is a forty-two-year-old married psychotherapist with extensive personal experience with psychedelic drugs. DMT is a powerful, short-acting psychedelic that occurs naturally in human body fluids, and is also found in many plants. Elena has read some Buddhism, but practices Taoist meditation.

She lies in a bed on the fifth floor of the University of New Mexico Hospital General Clinical Research Center. The clear plastic tubing that provides access to her vein dangles onto the bed. The cuff of a blood pressure machine is loosely attached to her other arm, and the tubing snakes its way into the back of a blinking monitor.

Within thirty seconds of the injection, she loses awareness of the room, and us in it. Besides myself, Elena's husband, who has just undergone a similar drug session, and our research nurse sit quietly by her side. I know from previous volunteers' reports that peak effects of intravenous DMT occur between two and three minutes after the injection, and that she will not be able to communicate for at least fifteen minutes, by which time most effects will have faded. Her eyes closed, she begins spurting out laughter, at times quite uproarious, and her face turns red. "Well, I met a living buddha! Oh, God! I'm staying here. I don't want to lose this. I want to keep my eyes closed to allow it to imprint itself. Just because it's possible!"

Elena felt great the next week. "Life is very different. A buddha is now always in the upper right-hand corner of my consciousness," says Elena. "All of what I have been working on spiritually for the last several years has become a certainty. Left hooks from the mundane world continue to come up and hit me, but the solidity of the experience anchors me, allows me to handle it all. Time stopped at the peak of the experience; now everyday time has slowed. The third stage, that of coming down from the peak, was the most important; if I had opened my eyes too soon I wouldn't have been able to do as much integrating of the experience as I have."

Two years later, Elena rarely takes psychedelics. Her most positive recollection of the DMT session was the "clarity and purity of the medicine." The most negative: "The absolute lack of sacredness and context." Many of the changes in her life, particularly a deepening shift from "thinking" to "feeling," were "supported" by the DMT session, but were underway before it, and continued after it.

Elena's experience, repeated by 10 to 20 percent of the volunteers in our psychedelic drug trials, represents the most gratifying and intriguing results of our work in New Mexico. My own interest in Buddhism and psychedelics meet in the most positive way in her DMT-induced "enlightenment experience."

Ours was the first new project in twenty-five years to obtain U.S. government funding for a human psychedelic drugs study. This scientific research was the result of eighteen years of medical and psychiatric training and experience. I also have been practicing Zen Buddhism for over twenty years. And it is in the molecule DMT where these two interests have finally merged.

There are important medical reasons to study psychedelic drugs in humans. The use of LSD ("acid") and "magic" mushrooms (which contain psilocybin) continues to climb. Understanding what psychedelics do to brain function, and how, will help treat short- and long-term negative reactions to them. Because there is some similarity of symptoms between psychedelic drug states and schizophrenia, psychedelic drug research also may shed new light on this devastating mental illness.

There are other reasons to study psychedelic drugs. Although less "medical," they do relate to health and well-being. Primary among them is the overlap between psychedelic and religious states. I was impressed by the "psychedelic" descriptions of intensive meditation practice within some Buddhist traditions. Because their scriptures did not mention drugs, and the states sounded similar to those resulting from psychedelic drug use, I suspected there might be a naturally occurring psychedelic molecule in the brain that was triggered by deep meditation.

I was led to the pineal gland as a possible source of psychedelic compounds produced under certain unusual mental or physical states. These conditions would include near-death, birth, high fever, prolonged meditation, starvation, and sensory deprivation. This tiny organ, the "seat of the soul" or "third eye" of the ancients, might produce DMT or similar substances by simple chemical alterations of the well-known pineal hormone melatonin, or of the important brain chemical serotonin. Perhaps it is DMT, released by the pineal, that opens the mind's eye to spiritual, or nonphysical, realities.

The pineal gland also held a fascination for me because it first becomes visible in the human fetus at forty-nine days after conception. This is also when the gender of the fetus is first clearly discernible. Forty-nine days, according to several Buddhist texts, is how long it takes the life force of one who has died to enter into its next incarnation. Perhaps the life-force of a human enters the fetus at forty-nine days through the pineal. And it may leave the body, at death, through the pineal. This coming and going would be marked by the release of DMT by the pineal, mediating awareness of these awesome events.

In addition to the scientific puzzle presented by the similarities between psychedelic and mystical consciousness, there were issues of healing that also drew me to both. The sense of there being "something greater" resulting from major psychedelic episodes led me to think that psychedelics might be helpful to people with psychological, physical, or spiritual problems. It seemed crucial to avoid the narrowness that often spoiled claims for the drugs' usefulness or dangers, and to hold a broad view. My emerging worldview resembled a tripod supported by biological (brain), psychoanalytic (individual psychology), and Eastern religious (consciousness and spirituality) legs. The first two legs were important in my decision to attend medical school. The third pushed me deeper into Buddhism.

Disheartened by the lack of spirit in medical training, I took a year's leave of absence from medical school and explored Zen in a series of retreats. Zen's emphasis on direct experience, its evenhanded approach to all mental phenomena encountered during meditation, and the importance of enlightenment all fit with my image of an ideal religious tradition. During my four-year psychiatric training, I helped found and run a meditation group affiliated with my long-standing Zen community. I was ordained as a lay Buddhist in the mid-1980s. This was the same year I trained in clinical psychopharmacology, learning to administer psychoactive drugs to human volunteers in controlled scientific studies.

The form our research in New Mexico took was a traditional biomedical one, monitoring effects of several DMT doses on blood pressure, temperature, pupil size, and blood levels of several chemicals indicating brain function. We recruited experienced hallucinogen users who were psychologically and medically fit. This was because they would be better able to report on their experiences, and less likely to panic or suffer longer-lasting side effects, than drug-inexperienced volunteers. Volunteers believed in the ability of psychedelics to help "inner work," and volunteered, at least in part, to use DMT for their personal growth.

Was there a spiritual aspect to the DMT experience? And, if so, was this helpful in and of itself? This was one of my deeper reasons for developing our DMT research program.

Supervising sessions is called "sitting," usually believed to come from "baby-sitting" people in a highly dependent and, at times, confused and vulnerable state. But, in our minds, Buddhist practice is as relevant a source for the term. Our research nurse and I did our best to practice meditation while with our volunteers: watching the breath, being alert, eyes open, ready to respond, keeping a bright attitude, and getting out of the way of the volunteer's experience. This method is very similar to what Freud called "evenly suspended attention," performed by a trained psychoanalyst who provided support by a mostly silent but present sitting by one's side. I experienced this type of listening and watching as similar to Zen meditation.

Another example of how psychedelic and Buddhist meditation converged was in the development of a new questionnaire to measure states of consciousness. Previous questionnaires measuring psychedelic drug effects were not ideal for many reasons. Some assumed that psychedelics caused nothing but psychosis, and emphasized unpleasant experiences. Other scales were developed using volunteers, sometimes ex-narcotic-addict prisoners, who were not told what drugs they were given or what the effects might be. I had always liked the Buddhist view of the mind being divided into the five *skandhas* ("heaps," "piles," or "aggregates") which, taken as a whole, give the impression of a personal self who experiences. These are the familiar "form," "feeling," "perception," "consciousness," and "volition." I looked into several guides to the Abhidharma literature, the Buddhist "psychological canon" with over a thousand years of use monitoring progress in meditation. It seemed that a *skandha*-based rating scale could provide an excellent basis for a neutral, descriptive understanding of psychedelic states.

I let it be known I was interested in talking with people who had taken DMT. Soon, the phone was ringing with people wanting to describe their experiences. Most of the nineteen people were from New Mexico and the West Coast, and nearly all were involved in some therapeutic or religious discipline. They were well-educated, articulate, and impressed with DMT's ability to open the door to highly unusual, nonmaterial states, which was greater than that of longer-lasting psychedelics like psilocybin or LSD. After completing these interviews, I decided to add a sixth *"skandha"* to the questionnaire, called "intensity," which helped quantify the nature of the experience.

We gave and analyzed this new questionnaire, the Hallucinogenic Rating Scale (HRS), almost 400 times to more than fifty people over four years. It is interesting to note that the grouping of questions using the *skandha* method gave more sensitive results in our DMT work than did a large number of biological measurements, such as blood pressure, temperature, or levels of certain chemicals in the blood.

Besides informing our style of sitting for and measuring responses to drug sessions, Buddhism helped make sense of the experiences people had in our relatively sparse but supportive environment. For many volunteers, even those with prior DMT use, the first high dose of intravenous DMT was like a near-death state, which in turn has been strongly linked to beneficial mystical experiences. Several were convinced they were dead or dying. Many had encounters with deities, spirits, angels, unimaginable creatures, and the source of all existence. Nearly all lost contact with their bodies at some point. Elena's case is a good example of an enlightenment experience—sounding identical to reports in the Buddhist meditative tradition—brought on by a high dose of DMT.

On one hand, a Buddhist perspective might hold all of these experiences to be equal. The matter-of-fact approach to nonmaterial realms in Buddhism provides firm footing for accepting and working with those experiences. It also does away with judging nonmaterial realms as better (or worse) than material ones—a tendency in some New Age religions. The experience of seeing and speaking to *deva*-like creatures in the DMT trance was just that: seeing and speaking with other beings. Not wiser, not less wise, and not more or less trustworthy than anyone or anything else.

On the other hand, how to meet head-on the volunteer who had a drug-induced enlightenment? Certify him or her as enlightened? Explain away by pharmacology the earth-shattering impact of the experience?

It was confusing. At first, it seemed as if a big dose of DMT was indeed transformative. As time elapsed, though, and we followed our volunteers for months and years, my perspective radically changed. While some, like Elena, had profoundly beneficial results from her participation, a small number of volunteers had frightening, negative responses that required some care afterward. Other, more subtle adverse effects also crept in (as may happen with Buddhist practice) in the form of increased self-pride—that is, a division into those with and without "understanding." In addition, "solving" problems while in an altered state—particularly common with high-dose psychedelic use—but then not putting the solution into practice, seemed to me worse than not even trying to work on the specific problem.

I have concluded that there is nothing inherent about psychedelics that has a beneficial effect, nor are they pharmacologically dangerous in and of themselves. The nature and results of the experience are determined by a complex combination of the drug's pharmacology, the state of the volunteer at the time of drug administration, and the relationship between the individual and the physical and psychological environment: drug, set, and setting.

The volunteers who benefited most from their DMT sessions were those who probably would have gotten the most out of any "trip"—drug or otherwise. Those who benefited least were those who were the most novelty-saturated. The most difficult sessions took place in combinations of two factors, the first being an unwillingness to give up the internal dialogue and body-awareness; and the second being uncertain or confusing relationships between the volunteer and those in the room at the time. Therefore, the "religious," "adverse," or "banal" effects resulting from drug administration depended more upon the person and what he or she and those in the room brought to the session, than on any inherent characteristic of the drug itself.

Thus, the problem with depending on one or several transformative psychedelic experiences as a practice is that there is no framework that suitably deals with everyday life between drug sessions. The introduction of certain Amazonian hallucinogenic plant-using churches into the West, with their sets of ritual and moral codes, may provide a new model combining religious and psychedelic practice.

In the last year of our work, a more difficult personal interplay of Buddhism and psychedelics appeared. This involved what might be described as a turf-battle developing between my Zen community and me. For years, I had been given at least implicit support to pursue my research by several members of the Zen community. These were senior students with their own prior psychedelic experiences. In the last year, I described our work to psychedelic-naive members of the community, who strongly condemned it. Formerly sympathetic students appeared pressured to withdraw any support for my studies. This concern was specifically directed at two aspects of our research. One aspect was a planned psychedelic-assisted psychotherapy project with the terminally ill, research that demonstrated impressive potential in the 1960s. That is, in patients who were having difficulty with the dying process, a "dry run" with a high-dose psychedelic session might ease the anguish and despair associated with their terminal illness. The other area of concern was the potential for adverse effects, both the obvious and more subtle ones previously described.

Scriptural and perceptual bases for this disapproval were given, in addition to community members' own and others' experiences. However, it appeared to me that the major concern was that it would be highly detrimental for them, as a Buddhist community, to associate Buddhism with drug use in any way. It appeared that those students who had their own psychedelic experiences (and had found them to stimulate their interest in a meditative life) had to close ranks with those who did not.

What I have experienced as the friction between disciplines is not uncommon in the world at large, and perhaps within the Buddhist community in particular. That is, is it "Buddhist" to give, take, or otherwise occupy oneself with psychedelics as spiritual tools?

Several research projects are being planned across the U.S., using psychedelics to treat intractable drug abuse—a condition with a high mortality rate if untreated. I understand Buddhist precepts to condone the use of "intoxicants" for medical purposes (e.g., cocaine for local anesthesia, narcotics for pain control). Whether or not a Buddhist who gives or takes a psychedelic "intoxicant" for the treatment of a medical condition faces similar criticism will be important to note. Complicating this case is the point that the psychological/spiritual effects of a properly prepared and supervised psychedelic session might be seen as curative.

In a final area of possible overlap, I believe there are ways in which Buddhism and the psychedelic community might benefit from an open, frank exchange of ideas, practices, and ethics. For the psychedelic community, the ethical, disciplined structuring of life, experience, and relationship provided by thousands of years of Buddhist communal tradition has much to offer. This well-developed tradition could infuse meaning and consistency into isolated, disjointed, and poorly integrated psychedelic experiences. The wisdom of the psychedelic experience, without the accompanying and necessary love and compassion cultivated in a daily practice, may otherwise be frittered away in an excess of narcissism and self-indulgence. Although this is also possible within a Buddhist meditative tradition, it is less likely with the checks and balances in place within a dynamic community of practitioners.

However, dedicated Buddhist practitioners with little success in their meditation, but well along in moral and intellectual development, might benefit from a carefully timed, prepared, supervised, and followed-up psychedelic session to accelerate their practice. Psychedelics, if anything, provide a view that—to one so inclined—can inspire the long hard work required to make that view a living reality.

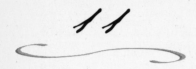

The Psychedelic
Vision at the
Turn of the
Millennium:
A Discussion with
Andrew Weil, M.D.

In August 1997, I organized a conference entitled The Psychedelic Vision at the Turn of the Millennium *for the annual meeting of the Association for Transpersonal Psychology, in Monterey, California. The first speaker to present his views was Andrew Weil, Clinical Professor of Internal Medicine at the University of Arizona School of Medicine and prolific author in the field of alternative medicine. Dr. Weil, who encountered hallucinogens as a student at Harvard University in the early 1960s, describes his initial experiences with mind-altering substances and the value he believes the powerful psychedelic vision has had in his own life and to our culture. The true significance of hallucinogens, he reminds us, is not to repeat the vision over and over, but to implement what one has learned from the experience into one's life for the purpose of personal and social change. Weil describes the extraordinary potential these compounds may have within the field of medicine as tools for learning, diagnosis and treatment.*

A. WEIL: I read *The Doors of Perception* in the summer of 1960 and then in that fall I entered Harvard as a freshman and was very eager to try mescaline as a result of reading that book. I had no idea, I had never heard of these substances, I had no experiences of any psychoactive substance other than alcohol, and in my naïveté, the first thing I did was go to my corner druggist and ask if he knew where I could get mescaline. He said that he had heard that there were experiments going on of trying to reproduce schizophrenia in the laboratory but he had no idea where you could get it. And I remember, I talked to several people, I asked my family doctor. I made the mistake of talking about it at the dinner table one night, and I saw the reactions it produced in my parents so I said nothing further. And then by coincidence that Fall, Aldous was at MIT as a visiting professor and gave a series of lectures, I think four lectures on visionary experience, which were broadcast on the Harvard radio station on Saturday afternoons. I listened to them entranced, those lectures that later became, I believe, *Heaven and Hell,* is that correct?

LAURA HUXLEY: No, I think that those lectures are part of a book called, *The Human Situation.*

A. WEIL: Well, they were very inspiring so I wrote a letter to Aldous Huxley. I think I sent it to him in care of MIT and he sent a handwritten letter back, giving me the name of a chemical company that he thought would sell mescaline. This was called Delta Chemical in New York. I wrote them a letter, this was in the pre-thalidomide days when there was not very much checking about who got what and they would indeed sell mescaline, but at about five times the price that it should be selling for, with no questions asked. I then heard that there was a professor named Leary who was interested in these substances. So I went over to see him and he said that he was sorry that I couldn't be in their experiments because he couldn't use undergraduates, but he said I should just keep checking and I could probably find it. I think I wrote back to Delta Chemicals and said, did they know anyone else who manufactured mescaline, and they gave me the names of three companies and they sent out these

forms that were fairly simple to fill out for using the drugs for investiga-
tional use. I mean this was in the innocent days and I found one of these
companies that was willing to sell mescaline and developed a nice relationship with them. It would arrive by UPS outside my dormitory, twenty-
four hours after I ordered it. So, I am very indebted to Aldous for the lead.

The first time I tried it, I tried it with one other friend of mine, and
there was a group of people in my freshman dorm who were interested in
it, but everybody was quite scared. I and this other fellow had volunteered
to try it first. It was not an ideal setting, with the two of us taking it with a
whole group of people sitting around, waiting to see what would happen.
It was on a Saturday afternoon and my set was so filled with anxiety that it
was about three or four hours before I felt anything at all. When I did feel
something, at the beginning it felt like alcohol intoxication; that was really
the only model I had for what an altered state was like. At the moment I
started to feel something the phone rang, and it was my mother calling
from Philadelphia, who never called on Saturdays. I mean it was an awkward conversation. She asked me about the weather and I said it was nice
and she said, "Why aren't you outside," and, "What are you doing?" and I
said I was just sitting around with some friends. She said, "I hope you are
not doing anything foolish like taking mescaline." I had mentioned the
word once about two months before. Mothers . . .

I said that I would talk to you about practicalities and my interest is,
"Okay, you have seen the psychedelic vision and you know, now—what do
you do with it?" You can see it over and over if you like, but it seems to me
the challenge is how do you translate it and what do you do with it. There
are a lot of people in our culture who have had this vision now, and our
concern is how is this going to be implemented. What can we do about it.

So again, I will talk very personally about this. Let me begin by just giving you some of the key elements of the particular vision that I experienced
as a result of psychedelic experimentation. The first, I think, is a sense of
wonder, of just wonder and awe at the universe, at life, at consciousness.
While that may seem simple, one of the things that has been very disap-
pointing to me and striking in my career in medicine and the sciences, is
the absence of that feeling on the part of many, if not most of my col-

leagues and I find that very dismaying. In fact, I even detect a strong feeling among some of the hard-core scientists that I went up against, that it is the business of science to do away with wonder. That science is seen as being able to roll back the mystery. I remember hearing Terence once say, he used an image which is terrific, that the bigger you build a fire and the more illumination it gives off, the more it makes you aware of the extent of the darkness beyond. I think that is very true, that fits with my experience and I think that is very much at odds with the scientific view, that the business of science is to do away with mystery. It seems to me that mystery is at the heart of existence and it is something that one experiences very profoundly as part of the psychedelic vision, whether it is the heavenly vision or the hellish vision. That has always been a very motivating force in my life. I think it has also kept alive my sense of curiosity. I am a very curious person and I check things out and I do it with this sense of wonder and it seems to me that is a very healthy attitude to have. Especially very healthy as a scientist and a physician. So, I have always tried to inspire that in people that I come into contact with, and in medical students, but I am very aware that I am up against a tremendous force in the opposite direction. It seems to me that is one thing that I try always to counter in my teaching, that comes directly from that psychedelic vision.

Another aspect of the psychedelic vision, for me, was the sense that anything is possible. That although there may be relative limits in the here and now, in some higher sense, there are no limits, that we live in a universe and that infinity and endless possibility are there. And again, I emphasize that this is a contrast because I think we live simultaneously in the three dimensional world where limitation exists and in some higher dimensional reality where it doesn't, so there is paradox there.

I will give you a very practical story about my experience of no limits. I wrote it down in a book that Lester Grinspoon edited on the psychedelic experience, but I will just repeat this for you because it has been for me a very meaningful model and one that has, again, motivated me in my work. This incident took place about 1970. I was living in rural Virginia, it was at the time that I was getting ready to write *The Natural Mind* and it was a period of great transition, when I had quit a government job and dropped out of medicine and was starting to meditate and do yoga and became a vegetarian. It was a time of great change in my life. Also, the political times in those days were both scary and very optimistic. One day in the spring of that year I took LSD with a group of friends, it was a perfect spring day and I was just in a wonderful state. I had been trying to start Hatha Yoga, as of a couple of months, and I had a lot of difficulty with some of the postures. The posture that I had the most difficulty with was the Plow, where you lie on your back and try to bend your feet down behind your head and touch the ground. I could get them down to about a foot from the ground and I would feel an excruciating pain in my neck. There was no progress at this, I had worked at it for about two months and I was on the point of giving up. I was twenty-eight, I decided I was too old and that my body was just out of shape and wasn't made for this. Well, in this LSD state I was just feeling so happy. I observed that my body felt completely elastic and springing and I thought, "Well gee, while I'm this way I ought to try doing the Plow." So I lay down and I was lowering my feet behind my head and I thought I had about a foot to go and they touched the ground. I couldn't believe it! And I kept raising them and lowering them and it was just, it was fabulous. The next day I tried to do it and I could get my toes to within a foot of the ground and there was excruciating pain in my neck, but there was a difference now. The difference was that I had seen that it was possible. And I don't think I would have believed that, I was on the point of giving up.

That experience of seeing that it was possible, even though it had now disappeared, motivated me to keep trying, and in the space of about three weeks I was able to do it. I think if I hadn't had that experience, I would have given up trying to do it. And to me that is a model for one aspect of what psychedelics can give you. It can give you a vision of possibility, but then it doesn't show you anything about maintaining that possibility. When the vision goes, the drug wears off, you are back where you were, you haven't learned anything but you have seen that something is possible. It is then up to you to figure out how to manifest the possibility. I think that sense of anything is possible has enabled me to accomplish a lot of things that I have done.

About three years ago my best friend from medical school was named Chief of Medicine at the University of Arizona by, again, total stroke of fate. He and our dean were a team at the University of Massachusetts, the two of them had been instrumental in getting Jon Kabat-Zinn's program set up at the University of Massachusetts. So when he arrived out in Arizona, he said, "Well now that you have friends in high places, what do you want to do?" I said, "Well, I would like to change all of medicine." And he said, "Well, how do you want to do that," and I said, "Here is what I would like to do," and I outlined the basis of this program in Integrative Medicine, which has now started and is in full swing. Our first doctor trainees are on board and—this is big stuff—the whole school is behind it. It is, I think, a model for medical education for the future and it is going to happen all over the country. And by the way, when people hear about it, I think the most common piece of feedback I get is people saying, "It's about time." It is long overdue, you know, and it is about time, but, I think if I didn't have that sense that anything is possible, I wouldn't have attempted anything of that sort. But I always do, I just have this sense of, "Why not?" and I think that comes directly from the psychedelic vision.

Another aspect of the psychedelic vision for me that has been very profound, is the sense that everything is alive or that at least, there is no distinction between what we call living and non-living. That there is some level on which everything is patterns of energy and that I have perceived that energy. I remember being in a canyon in Arizona in a psychedelic state and really being aware and able to see energy circulating in my hand, which was resting on a rock and to see that the energy in my hand was the same as the energy in the rock. That this was the same stuff, that everything is composed of basically the same stuff, which is in active movement. I think that sense has also led me to be very open to techniques and ideas in medicine that many of my colleagues find unable to fit in with their world views.

For instance, I have always been extremely interested in energy healing and all of the touch techniques. You look at my friend who is Chief of Medicine, Joe Alpert, a cardiologist; and he is a remarkably open person to be in the position of Chief of Medicine. As I said, he was a good friend of Jon Kabat-Zinn's and as a result of his association with our Program, his horizons have been greatly widened. But he said to me the other day, "You know you can talk to me about herbal medicine, I have no problem with osteopathic manipulation or acupuncture, but don't talk to me about homeopathy." He said, "I don't want to hear it," and this is the attitude of many. I think of all of the alternatives out there, homeopathy is probably the one that most pushes the buttons of the scientists, because it is the one that really challenges the materialistic paradigm. Here is a system of medicine based on giving people remedies that are so dilute that there is little chance that the molecules are present and Hahnemann, who invented this system said that he was liberating the spiritual essence of the drug in this way. He wasn't interested in a drug as a material substance, he was interested in it on the non-material level. Whether you want to call that the energy of the drug or the vibrational aspect of the drug or the spiritual aspect of the drug, you can not use that language in talking to medical doctors and scientists. It just enrages them.

For that reason I have deliberately made homeopathy one of the required subjects that we are teaching in the Program for Integrative Medicine. I have done that very deliberately because I think it is interesting to see what happens when you push all those buttons in an academic medical center. But my reason for doing that is exactly from my direct experience— from the psychedelic vision—of energy being the basis of everything, that it is possible to approach the human body on an energetic level and that may be a very valuable way of doing things. I want to see what happens there, if you try to look at this in a scientific way or try or are forced to develop a new conceptual paradigm to explain how therapies can interact with the human body. I want to push that envelope and see what happens.

I could go on in this vein but the main thing I want to leave you with is that for me, the challenge has been to translate these experiences that I've had in psychedelic states. I don't use psychedelics very frequently anymore. It is really a period of experimentation that was in my past, but my work is very actively derived from those experiences. It seems to me that the challenge in our culture is not to have this vision over and over again, it is really to see how the vision can be put into practice. How can you implement it into this sphere of life in which you are involved and produce change in that sphere, whatever it is. Mine happens to be medicine and that has been a big one to take on, as you can imagine, but for a variety of reasons it is very susceptible at the moment to being moved in a big way. The reasons, by the way, on a material level, are primarily economic.

Medicine is in enormous economic crisis today, it is really of its own making. It set out on a course of being very uncritically involved with technology and the dependence on technology is too expensive. At the same time it is up against this enormous worldwide, social, psychological shift among consumers who for a variety of reasons are moving toward natural things. These combined economic forces are irresistible. Medical institutions suddenly really have no choice but to move in this direction, but it is amazing to watch it all happen so fast. At any rate, I am very optimistic about the possibility for change there.

That reminds me of one other thing. I was interviewed very extensively in the past few months by a *New York Times* reporter, who was publishing some long feature, she is a woman in her mid-thirties who is a Harvard graduate, the daughter of two Harvard psychiatrists, I liked her very much and she is very thoughtful, very interesting and she wanted to read my whole body of work and asked lots of questions. She started asking me about the drug stuff and I said, "You really should read *The Natural Mind* first and then come back and talk to me." So she started *The Natural Mind* and she called up and said that she found it such a curious book; she said it seems so dated. I said, "What do you mean by dated?" and she said, "Well, it just seems like it is a product of another time." I said that, well, it was, but I said, "What do you mean by that?" She said, "Well, it is so optimistic." As I began talking to her about that actually I felt quite sad. She said that in her peers, her generation, going through college . . . the sense that you could change the world, is completely foreign to her, that it is so strange to read. In a sense, this makes me feel very sad and yet again I think that that optimism is something that for me derived from the psychedelic vision. I don't know whether her generation has not had that, but if younger people find that a dated view of reality, I feel very sorry for them. I think my sense of optimism is very much confirmed by what I see actually happening out there.

You know, I really do think the world is changeable and that all this can move quickly and astonishingly. I think also, even though change probably builds on slow incremental movements, that when it becomes perceptible sometimes the shifts are sudden. This is a popular view with Chaos Theorists. To point out an example that I have seen used; if you have a fish tank with fish and each day you are putting slightly more food in than the fish can eat, without knowing that one day you came in and the water is opaque and the fish are dead and floating on the surface. You wonder how could that be, what happened, but what happened was the result of very slow increments in which the flora was changed, the oxygen content of the water was changed. When it reaches a flip point, then there is this gross obvious change that seems to happen instantaneously. I think that is the way social change happens and world change happens as well. So, I think that doesn't spare you from doing the work day to day and putting it into action but then I think the movements can be very dramatic and sudden and amazing, so I remain extremely optimistic. And it just makes me very sad if that is true of the generation younger than me. So, I will stop there and let you comment.

CHARLES GROB: Thank you, Andy. It's certainly good to have you here at a meeting like this, talking about these issues. Clearly you are in the public eye, as a spokesperson for the field of alternative medicine, which is having an enormous impact on how people are viewing health and are viewing what they need to do to ensure their own health. You are certainly having an impact being right out there, center stage. What is also quite extraordinary is looking at your own history and in a sense, where your early vision was acquired. I think this is one of the attributes of the psychedelics which often goes unacknowledged; the power with which they endow individuals with a vision that often takes them forward in their lives. Even individuals who haven't taken psychedelics in years or in decades will often trace back pivotal decisions they have made to those early experiences. I think it is really gratifying to see you, particularly now in your position of prominence, very willing to speak of such early experiences.

It is also quite fascinating to examine the medical profession in flux. One of our institutions that seems to be so impervious to even the slightest change, is now moving at a rapid rate. I wonder at what point might our profession start to open up to the potentials that psychedelics might have in terms of helping us understand health, understand illness and understand new methods to intervene. Sometimes I, in my wildest of optimistic visions, imagine a field of psychedelic medicine devoted to studying this phenomenon, a phenomenon that has gone virtually ignored by Western medicine. But if you look back on the roots of our healing structures, that which we inherited from our ancestors, we see that much of early, very early so-called primitive medicine was on the Shamanic healing model, which often used altered states acquired through one method or another to facilitate healing; either through the healer getting inside into the malady of the person and implementing energetic changes, or the patient him or herself entering an altered space to facilitate a process of healing. If we look to the future and anticipate an evolution of our medical systems, might it be possible even to imagine a role that psychedelics might play? Even a role that is accepted and valued?

A. WEIL: Actually that reminds me, I left out one very important component of the psychedelic vision, which for me was the real experience that external reality can be changed by changing internal reality. That is, that by doing something in here, everything out there changes and I think that has enormous relevance for medicine. I will give you another personal experience. I think this was on a different occasion than that one I told you about with the yoga experience, but it was again with LSD. I had had a lifelong allergy to cats and didn't like cats. If I touched a cat and then touched my face my eyes would itch and swell, and if a cat licked me I got hives where they licked, so I always stayed away from cats. One day in an LSD state, when I was feeling very centered, a cat jumped in my lap and I just decided, well, I was going to enjoy the cat. So I played with the cat extensively, I had no allergic reaction and I have never had one since. That to me was a very powerful experience, how something that I thought was a lifelong pattern could change in an instant as a result of a change in internal reality.

I have one other to contribute, this one I have not written about but it is even more impressive. I had very fair skin as a child and was always told I couldn't get tan. We used to go down to the Jersey beaches in the summer and I remember endless sunburns with sheets of skin peeling off, this was in the days by the way, when what we used for suntan lotion were products that probably magnified the sun reaching your skin. But this is something I just accepted about myself; that I couldn't get tan, that my skin would peel and that was always my experience. At this same period in 1970 when I was making all these changes in my life; I decided that this is something that has got to change. I remember, again with psychedelics, for the first time I lay naked in the sun and exposed my whole body to sun, and lo and behold, my skin got tan for the first time in my life and it has ever since.

Those have been very remarkable experiences: the sense of anything is possible, that there are no limits, at least in the ideal world, and that the key to changing external reality and reactions to the environment lies in internal transformations. When I work with patients, especially patients who have chronic pain or chronic illnesses, even though I may not know how to do it, I think it is important to give them a sense that this is changeable and that they should keep experimenting. My general sense is that the real change is at the level of consciousness. If these tools were available to us as practitioners, I could see a lot of potential uses there and not just in psychiatric medicine, which is where it has been talked about the most, but especially in physical medicine.

I think you could take people with severe allergies, for example, and give them a series of experiences with decreasing doses of the drug to teach them how to unlearn an allergy and maybe in similar ways you could teach people how to unlearn chronic pain or to unlearn musculoskeletal problems or digestive problems. I could see great potential use for it.

C. GROB: I think it's good to hold this concept that anything is possible, a sense that even structures that we feel are too resistant to change, can change. To hold an optimistic vision of what may be possible. I think we are beginning to see examples that the realization may be more accessible than we had thought.

For example, no one really anticipated the collapse of Eastern Europe, the way it happened with such rapidity and in such an overwhelming manner. I think we are going to see in medicine simply more receptivity. The public at large wants alternative perspectives, alternative approaches, the very notion of putting forward a program for training practitioners in alternative medicine at a prestigious medical school, ten years ago, would have been unheard of. That would have been a pipe dream of the widest magnitude and here it's already starting to happen. So, I think in a sense what we need are visions such as this and a sense of surety that with time and persistence change is feasible. I think this is really a powerful example for us to hold and also for us to carry with us as we take the visions that we have for the future, but also with realization that change is possible. Dennis, do you have some comments here?

DENNIS MCKENNA: Yes I do, I think that Andy makes the good point, that psychedelics can be important in individuals' lives in terms of orienting them to a wider vision or be an influence in terms of directing people. I think psychedelics ultimately are something that you come to as an individual. The challenge that we face is trying to relate our own individual experience and its influence in our own lives to the greater society, and ultimately beyond society to our species' fate. This is where the challenge lies, trying to reconcile these two, because the way that at least our western society is structured, there are no paradigms for joining these two. In fact, societies seem mostly set up to discourage this kind of self discovery and to repress it by legislative means if necessary, but by whatever means. It is not something that is encouraged. I think that one of the biggest challenges for the next millennium is, how are we going to take our own individualistic psychedelic visions or inspirations and try to diffuse those into a larger society. This is always the problem.

As Andy has said earlier, now that you have the vision, what do you do with it and how do you somehow give expression to it in the way you live and the way that society operates. I think that is really the challenge. I am optimistic too, it must be that optimism is infectious because I think there are a lot of discouraging things going on but overall I think that trends are in the right direction.

L. HUXLEY: I would like to say one thing. Andy has given me, I think all of us, a great hope that one of these visionary common sense ideas might become true one of these days. I think that in a conscious society, a great doctor would say to his patient, look here, I am going to try to do my best for you but I can do very little. But I have one little bit of news, you can do a lot for yourself. Maybe that is going to happen because of you.

D. MCKENNA: I would like to ask Andy, do you see psychedelics as a potential diagnostic tool for physicians, being used much in the same way that ayahuasca for instance, would be in tradition settings?

A. WEIL: That's a very interesting question. We have twelve core subjects in the Integrative Medicine Program that the physicians are learning and we have recruited faculty of the whole University of Arizona as well as outside to develop these courses. One of the courses is called *The Art of Medicine* and this is all material that is not usually taught in medical schools; one aspect of this is intuition. I have always maintained that all diagnosis was based on intuition and that all of the great diagnosticians that I have met have been highly intuitive, although they may not have recognized that themselves. I think that the diagnostic tests that we do can be used to confirm or discard hunches that you form intuitively. But a problem in our educational system is that not only is intuition not rewarded, actually students are actively penalized for using intuition and not relying on objective data. And that has gotten even worse with the whole medical malpractice situation because now, with the great fear of litigation, there is more and more emphasis on not doing anything unless you have objective numerical data to support what you do. So, I am very much interested in how you train intuition in people and I could imagine a future world in which psychedelics were available for that, they could be used in a way to become more aware. Everybody is intuitive, but most of us aren't trained to pay attention to it or to act on it and I think that is the challenge. I could definitely see drugs being used in that way.

AUDIENCE QUESTION: Your talk made me think about three different kinds of people or three different kinds of situations, I am not quite sure how to say it but, there are people who have taken psychedelics early in their lives or careers and kicked the visions into their lives, there are people who are involved in spiritual practices in which the use of psychedelics is an ongoing thing and there are people who take psychedelics over and over again and don't seem to do very much into bringing it into their lives. Have you thought about what accounts for the differences among those three kinds of people?

A. WEIL: I haven't. I will add, by the way, a fourth category, which is people who have had the vision without ever using psychedelics. And they can either take it into their lives or not, as well. No, I haven't thought about that, I don't know. I don't know what accounts for that.

AUDIENCE QUESTION: My comment might be a good follow up to that. My experience started with spontaneous visions as a teenager and then into meditation and then occasional use of psychedelics and then a lot more meditation, long retreats which seemed to duplicate the psychedelic experience through natural meditative practices. And then, going into medicine and psychiatry and now six years of psychoanalytic training. I think the basic ego strength of the user before the psychedelic experience or the spontaneous ego experience is a big factor in whether you bring this vision into the world or not. We are getting into the realm of psychiatry and a lot of these issues may have to be dealt with, with a dialogue between internal medicine and psychiatry as well as alternative medicine. In many ways psychiatry may be behind the boat, but it may be the future of how we integrate. How do we bring forth the natural healing abilities of the unconscious mind into our personal lives and bring out those visions that are within us into manifestation in helping the world with its problems?

A. WEIL: That makes me think of several things; first is that the first time that I took mescaline in my freshman year, I really had minimal experience because I think I had so much anxiety about it. I took it again about a month later and had what certainly felt to me like a mystical experience and it was very overwhelming. But I think when I came out of it, some part of me knew that if I followed through with the implications of it I was not going to go through college and medical school. I kind of shut that all off and it wasn't until I was probably out of medical school, beginning to do an internship, that I began to experiment with psychedelics again and recover that. I think if at that point I would have pursued a psychedelic career I would have not gotten my medical degree and not done what I now do. So that makes me somewhat cautious about young people and that is one thing that I might tell young people; there may be an appropriate time in life to do this and that maybe it is worth waiting a certain period.

I can't imagine what would have happened to me if I would have discovered these drugs when I was in high school, for example. Another thought that I have is to what you said about psychiatry and medicine; I think this is one of the great tragedies of modern medicine and is really part of the legacy of Descartes. There are people who say that if western civilization took one wrong turn, it was with Descartes; certainly the split between psychiatry and medicine is in that Cartesian tradition. I think it is very unfortunate. I am doing what I can to repair that. I was asked to give psychiatry grand rounds at the University of Arizona a few months ago and to my delight, they were very unhappy that they had been left out of the Integrative Medicine Program and wanted to know how they could participate. So, I have definitely opened a dialogue with the psychiatry department. Even if they just want to get in on a level of doing research, that is fine. I would like to involve them much more. The concept behind psychiatry—the word means soul doctoring—I can't imagine anything more important, especially if you feel as I do, that much if not all of disease originates on the nonphysical level and then eventually manifests on the physical level. And yet, it is so ironic that of all of the medical specialties, psychiatry is the one that is most mired in materialism and sees all disorders of consciousness as being the result of brain biochemistry, when it could just as well be the other way around. And that all therapy is giving people drugs and if a psychiatrist is treating a person who develops a physical problem they are referred to an internist and if an internist has a patient who is believed to have an emotional problem, they are referred to a psychiatrist and there is no conversation there. That is a big problem, it is something very wrong with medicine today, and something that we are trying to fix.

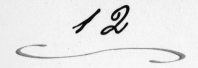

Making Friends
with Cancer
and Ayahuasca

Donald M. Topping, Ph.D.

The potential for hallucinogens to be applied to the treatment of medical illness has largely gone unexplored. Anecdotal accounts, particularly in the case of plant hallucinogens, however, do provide exciting leads for future research applications. Donald Topping, Professor Emeritus of Linguistics at the University of Hawaii, shares his story of how his metastatic colon cancer went into remission following several encounters with the Amazonian plant hallucinogen concoction, ayahuasca. Dr. Topping's remarkable experience with the legendary medicine of the tropical rain forest provides tantalizing clues of what we may have yet to learn from the extraordinary pharmacopoeia provided by Nature.

UNTIL SEVERAL YEARS AGO, I never dreamed that I would be writing about two subjects that are both generally considered taboo. One of these is cancer. We avoid talking about cancer—"the Big C"—because it reminds us of our fears of mortality and pain. When a friend or colleague is rumored to have cancer, we avoid the topic or speak in whispers about it.

138

For entirely different reasons, people talk in hushed tones about ayahuasca—the visionary brew from South America. The Drug Enforcement Administration—the grand arbiter of all psychoactive chemicals in America—is responsible for this taboo, as it has classified DMT, one of the brew's constituents, as a Schedule I drug, thereby rendering it illegal and nearly unavailable for medical, psychological, neurological, and spiritual research. Since I now enjoy the privileges of being a recently retired person and a friend of cancer and ayahuasca, I can speak freely about them both. I say "friend" because that is the way I now view my relationship with them.

My connection with cancer probably started with my birth seventy years ago, which sent me into the world with a genetic blueprint determined, at least in part, by ancestors on both sides of my family who had died of metastasized colorectal cancer. If there is any validity to the genetic predilection theory, I was directly in line for a firsthand experience with cells running amok to form tumors.

And that is precisely what happened to me twelve years ago, when I was first diagnosed with cancer of the colon. Since I felt great, I had doubts about the accuracy of the diagnosis, and I requested to see the biopsy along with a pathologist. Sure enough, with the aid of a microscope, I saw the little cells, all bunched up like globs of red mud. How did that happen? I wondered.

Immediate surgery was the prescription of the day, but I begged off temporarily in order to experiment with natural healing. The surgeon and I agreed on a four-month timetable, during which I followed a naturopathic regimen: microdoses of various substances, a vegetarian diet, visualizations, and plenty of rest and exercise. After this period, the second biopsy revealed no cancer cells, and I was overjoyed.

My surgeon seemed disappointed, and he asked for another biopsy in two weeks, to which I agreed. This time around, he was able to dig up some more tissue with cancer cells, and he convinced me that I should have the surgery. I did, and I was told five years later that I had been "cured" through the wonders of surgery.

All went well until September 1996, when a routine physical exam revealed that my CEA (carcinoembryonic antigen) count—an indicator of carcinogen activity—was up. Another blood test shortly thereafter showed the CEA count going up rapidly. Further exams were conducted, during which two suspicious-looking dark shadows were seen on the right lobe of my liver. A biopsy was soon performed on the tissue taken from the shadowed area. The verdict from the pathologist was "the Big C."

Having lost a grandfather and father to metastatic liver cancer, I was seriously concerned over this new development. What to do? A preliminary conference with one of the oncologists said that surgery might be a possibility, provided there were no other tumors in my vital organs or lymph glands. That meant further exams.

While waiting for the results, I went to the University of Hawaii's medical library for information on liver cancer. I was referred to the "bible" on oncology, a two-volume tome titled *Cancer: Principles and Practices of Oncology (1989)*, edited by Vincent T. DeVita, Jr. Turning to Section 3: "Treatment of Metastatic Cancer to the Liver," by John E. Niederhuber and William D. Ensminger, I was confronted with the following sobering paragraph:

"The spread of malignant cells from a primary tumor to the liver and their growth therein carry a grave prognosis for the patient. While these metastatic liver tumors may be the first evidence of the progression of a patient's cancer, and often—especially in colorectal cancer—are the only tumors detected, they almost always signal widespread dissemination of the malignancy. Despite improvements in early detection of liver metastases, new drug development, improved surgical techniques for resection, and innovative targeted therapies, most patients will not survive." (p. 2201)

The remainder of the chapter was devoted to sustaining that dismal prognosis. In a word, the future looked pretty grim. Until, that is, I began to seek information on alternative therapies. I turned first to Andrew Weil, M.D., who recommended the following regimen: have the tumor surgically removed, if possible; start taking microdoses of maitake mushroom extract; and read Michael Lerner's *Choices in Healing*.

While waiting for my mail-order purchases of maitake extract and Lerner's book to arrive, I had further meetings with surgeons, who were not exactly reassuring. I was told by one that my chances for survival were around 25–30 percent. Another put my odds at under 15 percent, once the risks of the surgical procedure itself were factored into the formula. I guessed that they, too, had read DeVita's cancer bible. They also advised me that, assuming surgery was possible, I should follow it up with a year of fairly heavy chemotherapy in order to kill off any remaining cancer cells (along with the majority of the healthy ones) that were floating around in my bloodstream.

When Lerner's book arrived in the mail, I sat down and read through its six hundred plus pages as rapidly as possible. At the same time, I began to take the maitake extract and to prepare myself both physically and mentally for the surgery and chemotherapy. During this period, I began to explore literature on other alternative therapies, including Essiac, macrobiotic diets, Reiki, and coffee enemas. At least these treatments offered more hope and encouragement than the oncologist's bible did.

On November 26, 1996, I entered the hospital and my surgeon (aptly named Dr. Payne) removed the right half of my liver. During the following five days, I was attached to several catheters, one of which shot morphine directly into my spine. It was not until my discharge from the hospital that I realized how badly my body had been assaulted, not just by the surgeon's knife but also by a mixture of drugs whose effects are considered unavoidable collateral damage of the invasive surgery. The thought of further assaulting my body with chemotherapy was frightening.

Sometime during my painful recovery from the operation, I remembered having read something about the healing properties of ayahuasca. Since it had seemed unlikely that I would visit the Amazon, and I wasn't particularly interested in a psychedelic experience, I hadn't given it much thought at the time. Still, the memory lingered in the recesses of my mind, which was still reeling from the physical and psychic wounds of major surgery—the outcome of which was still dubious.

Three weeks after the surgery, I went to an appointment with my oncologist, who proposed that I begin with the chemotherapy treatment immediately. When I told him that I had decided against it because I did not believe that further assault on my body would be beneficial, he seemed miffed, perhaps even insulted. When I mentioned my plan to follow a program of alternative therapies, he snickered but then wished me well.

My Initial Workings with Santo Daime

In early April 1997, I heard rumors of a group that was working with ayahuasca on the Big Island of Hawaii. I began to make inquiries, which led me to a young man who had been with the group for several experiences, or "works," as they are called in the Santo Daime religion of Brazil. When we met at my house one evening, the man talked non-stop for over three hours about the sacrament and its psychic and physical healing properties. As I listened, I grew intrigued. I soon concluded that I needed to have this experience, to see for myself if the accounts I had read and heard were true. Could this really be a curative experience, or was it just another psychedelic trip?

A few weeks later, I learned that there would be a works on the Big Island and that I could join the group. I readily accepted, even though I was still in a weakened condition from the surgery. This was to be my introduction to ayahuasca.

The group met in the late afternoon on an isolated knoll where a devotee of the Santo Daime had built a house, consisting of a large hexagonal room with several smaller rooms on the side. (I later learned that the hexagon is an important symbol within the Santo Daime religion.) About sixty people from all over Hawaii, most of whom had participated in Daime works before, had gathered for the event. We were all dressed in white (as required), and when the time came to begin, we took our seats in chairs that had been arranged in two semicircles facing each other, men on one side and women on the other. It dawned on me, much to my disappointment, that I was embarking on a very structured group experience. It wasn't at all what I had anticipated from my limited reading on the way ayahuasca is traditionally used by shamans in the Amazon. Nevertheless, I entered the experience with hope, as well as apprehension. The residual pain from the surgery reminded me why I was there.

I will not describe the Santo Daime rituals that I participated in during the two successive nights of the works. Those rituals have been described at length elsewhere (de Alverga 1996; Carvalho 1997). Rather, I will focus on my own experience, for which, as it turns out, I was unprepared. My only frame of reference was my limited experiences with LSD, mushrooms, and mescaline during the 1960s, and none of these psychoactive experiences had been associated with healing. I wanted to discover what it was about ayahuasca that led to the claims of its ability to heal and to teach.

After some preliminary church rituals, we lined up to each take our first cup of the brew just after sundown. A second dose would be given about two and a half hours later. Within twenty minutes, I began to feel a rippling effect coursing throughout my body. As I looked around the room, I noticed that many of the others were shifting restlessly in their chairs, trying to sing the church chants in Portuguese. I began to wonder if I had made the right decision.

Then, all of a sudden, the plant grabbed hold of me and led me on a long trip into another reality, one that I was totally unprepared for. As I closed my eyes, images—if they can be called such—began racing at an every-increasing speed before me. Swirls of colors, forms, textures, and sounds simply overpowered me to the point that I became immobile. Like many others before me, no doubt, I became somewhat frightened. What had I let myself in for?

When I opened my eyes, the phantasmagoria of forms vanished, and I saw myself in the same room with the others, most of whom were moving their lips to the songs being sung by the Brazilian leaders from the Santo Daime. I closed my eyes again, and immediately the images returned with surging intensity. They seemed to be trying to enter the deepest recesses of my body and soul. I found myself thinking, hey, this isn't much fun.

Following a period of initial disorientation, I was able to regain my focus on what had brought me to this medicine in the first place. I was a condemned man; the oncologists and their bible had told me that my chances of survival were slim. I had come to ayahuasca for a second opinion. That is when I began to let go and let the plant do its thing—and I began to get my first glimpse into the incredible, stunning world of ayahuasca. There was no going back now. There was nothing to do but let it happen.

As others have reported seeing, I saw plants, serpents, birds, and jaguar-like animals soaring, swirling, twisting, and racing at almost lightning speed throughout my entire system, as though they were exploring a new habitat. At first, they didn't pay any attention to me, even though I tried to stop them long enough to have a closer look. Before long, however, one of them raced up to me, paused momentarily, and then rushed off as though it had urgent business somewhere else. Then others came up to my face and did the same thing. There was no time for any communication between myself and the things that I was seeing. It was as though they wanted to take an inventory of who I was and what was going on inside me before they were ready to talk.

After a while (one loses track of time with ayahuasca), the figures began to slow down and fade somewhat in intensity. I was coming down, much against my will. My questions—whatever they were—had not yet been answered. At that moment, the Daime leader gave the signal to line up for the second dose of the brew. I took my place in the line.

Many of the group of sixty people had already been purged through vomiting, but I was not yet among them. As the second wave of ayahuasca ripples came over me, I felt much more relaxed. This time, I wanted to talk to the animals, if only they would talk to me. As though on cue, the racing figures began to stop by, look at me, and smile before darting off into their world again. Then, all of a sudden, I saw a deep, black void—nothing but darkness, which stayed in place for what seemed like minutes. All of the flashes, colors, and forms disappeared while the blackness hovered over me. I sensed that it was death, making its statement: "Yes, I'm here, too, part of the system—but I'm not so bad, so don't be afraid." In a short while, the darkness began to fade slowly and a kaleidoscopic frenzy ran its course until the brew and I both were exhausted. I returned to my friend's house for a long but fitful sleep.

The following evening, the group of sixty gathered again for a second session, which I entered with much less trepidation, hoping for more insights from the plant. That proved to be a false hope, perhaps because the plant had nothing more to tell me. Nevertheless, during the second trip, I again felt the presence of the plant racing throughout my body, peeking and poking into every nook and cranny in search of something to work on, to straighten out, to put back in order, to polish. There was a definite presence, with similar shapes, colors, and sounds, as on the previous night. But, unlike the first time, there was no message; the plant was just busy doing its work.

Several months passed before my next experience with ayahuasca. In the interim, I continued on my program of vegetarian food and Chinese herbs, which seemed to help. I was gradually regaining my weight and strength, while the scars and soreness of the surgery were slowly healing. I wanted to work with ayahuasca again, to determine whether my first experience had been delusional or not, and to see if the plant had any new insights for me.

Soaring to New Heights of Consciousness

By good fortune, I met a person who had studied with *ayahuasqueros* in Peru. When I told him what I was seeking, he agreed to lead me and four others through a private session. This time, the set and setting were entirely different from those of the structured Santo Daime. After bathing in warm, blue ocean water, we drove up to the end of a mountain road and hiked to an isolated spot on a small plateau deep in the Wai'anae Mountains of O'ahu. The setting, called Pupukea Highlands, was engulfed in lush foliage with an unobstructed view of the Pacific Ocean in two directions—in itself, an invitation for spirits to enter.

Our group was small, and we shared a common set: all of us had learned to respect the plant and its powers. We arrived at our spot in time to arrange our spaces before nightfall. By candlelight, we practiced deep breathing and toning exercises in preparation for taking the brew. Then, in ceremonial fashion, our guide blew tobacco smoke over the sacramental brew before offering some to each of us. Soon after, he extinguished the candles, reminding us, "The plant knows what it's doing." The isolation, silence, and darkness of the moonless night were awesome.

I positioned myself comfortably on the ground, my back against the trunk of a large paper-bark tree. Feeling very calm and relaxed, I closed my eyes and waited for the plant to go to work. Once again, after about fifteen minutes, I began to notice the now-familiar rippling wave effect. This time, however, the rippling accelerated into full-blown turbulence. The plant was loose, and it was wildly racing around, exploring its new environment. I felt as though a caged animal had been released inside me and it was having the time of its life.

As the images and shapes began to appear, they had an air of joy and exuberance. The serpents were smiling, the jaguars laughing, and the giant birds were swooping down, caressing me with their outstretched wings. A parade of persons, both known and unknown, streamed by, each of them smiling and reaching out to touch me, telling me by look that they loved me. As the serpents and plants twisted and flashed before me, I sensed they were reassuring me that they had checked everywhere inside me and that everything was okay. As the evening went on, this cycle kept repeating. Images would come directly towards me at breakneck speed, smiling and laughing, then veer off for another tour of my entire system. I heard myself chuckling softly under the starlit sky.

Where was the darkness that I had experienced before? Where was Mr. Death? I wondered. Then, as though the plant had heard my question, I saw the void. Only this time, it seemed to be peeping through a montage of vibrant colors and forms, as if to say, "I'm still here, don't worry. It's not time for me yet." And then it faded away. As evening turned into night and morning, I saw the images slowing down and gradually fading away, almost reluctantly, it seemed. We—the plant and I—sure had a good time together that night.

If ayahuasca could talk in words, I'm sure it would have told me during that first trip to Pupukea, "Take this energy that I'm giving you, and run with it. Latch on to one of the animals and go for the ride. There is nothing preventing you from soaring to new heights of consciousness and life." That was the message I got that first night in the Pupukea Highlands.

About one month after that memorable night, I revisited the Pupukea

Highlands for another ayahuasca session, this time with a different group of six people. I was eager for a repeat experience, another exciting exploration, and some reassurance from the plant—but that was not to be.

This time, it was raining, which restricted our space to the area inside a makeshift tent. We followed the same procedures as in the previous experience, breathing, toning, and ceremonially ingesting the brew. I lay down and waited for the action to begin. This time, the onset of the rippling was much more gradual, and it never reached the intensity of the previous trip. The images were there—birds, serpents, plants, and people—but they were much less energetic, almost blasé. They seemed to be telling me, "We've already been this route, and we told you what we found. Let's try something new." I realized that I had entered the experience with a programmed agenda, and the plant responded as though it were obliged. I could now see the value of trusting the plant to take the lead.

Approximately two weeks after that second session, I went for my next scheduled visit with the oncologist. He greeted me warmly, congratulating me on the results of my blood test the week before. It showed that my CEA count was not just normal; it was below normal! When he asked me what I had been doing to bring that about, I asked him if he had ever heard of ayahuasca. He hadn't, but as soon as I mentioned that it is a medicinal plant that has been used for centuries in the Amazon by shamans and healers, his response was exactly what one might expect from a physician trained in Western allopathic medicine. He raised his eyebrows and shrugged his shoulders, and I could almost hear him thinking to himself, "Where did this nut come from, anyway?" He ended that office visit with the pronouncement, "You're one of the lucky few."

Lucky? Perhaps so. But to dismiss my recovery against such hopeless odds as nothing but luck struck me as a very insular, unscientific viewpoint. In contrast to such skepticism, I have become an enthusiastic friend of ayahuasca. I decided not only to continue treating my body and my spirit with ayahuasca, but also to learn what I could about this marvelous plant medicine. In the process, I have discovered that my experience with ayahuasca and cancer is not unique. I keep hearing of other persons from different parts of the world who have had similar experiences. Some of these accounts have been reported to me by word of mouth, others in literature. There are too many reports to dismiss them all as merely chance.

Understanding Ayahuasca

After the first segment of this article was published in the *MAPS Bulletin* (1998, VIII:3), I received letters, e-mails, and telephone calls from many interested persons. Some were struggling to find cures for cancer, while others merely had a healthy curiosity about the vine. Their response took me by surprise and pushed me to explore further thoughts about the role of ayahuasca and what I believe has been happening with me. Many people are interested in knowing how it works. Frankly, so am I. Due to the absence of any definitive, clinically validated explanations, I will try to share my thoughts and insights, as provided by the vine and refined through discussions I've had with fellow travelers here and there.

Before sharing these thoughts, I need to state very clearly that I am not championing ayahuasca as a miracle cure for cancer or anything else. I am simply relating my own story and my sense of what is happening with me. At this point, my story is best taken as another anecdote in the growing body of lore surrounding the vine. Nonetheless, let me say that the original diagnosis that I had liver cancer was made in September 1996. Three years later, I am still healthy and the cancer appears to be in complete remission. And as I approach my seventieth year, I can honestly say that I have never felt better, aside from a couple of aching joints, reminders of my rough and tumble days. People often comment that I look particularly healthy and ask what I am doing to look that way. To some of these people, I explain that I have changed my diet to vegetarian foods, I exercise regularly, and I have all but stopped drinking alcoholic and caffeinated beverages—and that seems to satisfy them. To others, who seem ready to understand, I more frankly attribute my health to the vine.

Several ayahuasca researchers (notably J. Mabit, R. Grove, and J. Vega, 1995) have suggested that the vine appears to work in three domains: psychological, spiritual, and organic. My experience confirms this notion, although the distinction between psychological and spiritual is not as clearly defined for me as that between spiritual and organic. Perhaps that is because my initial use of ayahuasca was prompted by my quest to restore my physical health. Nevertheless, the psychological and spiritual dimensions have played an important, albeit a more subtle, role in my recovery.

Catalyzing Psychological Change

I experienced a most profound psychological change during my first experience, when I encountered death in the form of a soft, deep, dark void. I had been preoccupied with thoughts about my impending death—as predicted by my physician and the data. Interestingly, the vine put that fear to rest straight away. The clear message was that death is always present, but it is nothing to be feared. It is there, along with all the other forces and elements of nature. Death happens. Stating these obvious facts in words sounds trite. However, when the vine reveals such things, the impact is far more profound.

Among other psychological insights, I have been gifted with lessons on the relative importance of things in life. For example, during my fourth or fifth session, I saw a gallery of assorted clocks and watches, dozens if not hundreds of them, moving as though in a shooting gallery, with the minute and hour hands going rapidly in a counterclockwise direction. I interpreted this vision as a commentary on my preoccupation with time and my fear of running out of it before I could accomplish all my goals. The vine seemed to be saying, "OK, if that bothers you, let's make time run backwards." The revelation came to me that "time" is something that humans view as a commodity to be measured, valued, saved, wasted, and sold. In ayahuasca reality, time simply does not matter. Like death, time is always present, and living each day fully means much more than racking up achievements.

I have read that for others, including some drug addicts, ingestion of the vine tends to result in profound psychological processing, including letting go of one's ego and confronting the demon within, as the light illuminates the dark corners of the psyche. Some have reported this to be a difficult experience. Although I have not had this type of psychic encounter, I think I understand the process. Interacting with ayahuasca seemingly leaves little room for ego control, and the probing lights of the vine leave no dark corners in which demons can hide.

Illuminating the Spiritual Realm

The spiritual aspects of my ayahuasca experiences are even more difficult to describe and define. Not having been a spiritual type since my adolescent disillusionment with Christianity, I did not approach ayahuasca with any spiritual expectations. My sole mission had been to restore my physical health, which I naively believed to exist independently of my spiritual self. Ayahuasca persuaded me that I was wrong. How did this come to pass?

During ayahuasca-induced visions, I saw and head some astonishing things that have changed my perceptions and understanding of the forces at work in my universe. Plants often morphed into animals, and vice versa. In the dim shadows of the forest at night, the surrounding plants became vigorously alive, gently pulsating and moving toward me as though to join together with me. While there was nothing that suggested a singular deity, there was an unmistakable presence of a force that permeated the entire experience, linking my body with my inner self and with my entire surroundings: the others in the group, the plants, the air, and the stars and beyond.

At the onset of my visions, I have experienced waves of varicolored light separating into twisting, undulating ribbons of energy, at times resembling serpentine creatures, switching back and forth from plant to animal form, all the while emitting sounds that I can only describe as a rapid sequence of high-pitched chirps. Once, I tried to follow these upward-spiraling ribbons of light to see how far they would lead me into the infinite darkness. I soared upward, as though riding a comet's tail, until the ribbons split off, forming arcs that veered off in a trajectory that circled back to begin the cycle again. I began to see these ribbons as the energy force that unites everything—the life force, or spirit, of the living and dead—past, present, and future.

Organic Purification Rites

For myself, the organic or physical aspects of the ayahuasca experience have been easier to track and describe, perhaps because I began my relationship with the plant seeking the restoration of my health. My view of cancer, however unscientific, comes largely from having looked at my own cancerous cells under an electron microscope in the company of a pathologist. Quite clearly, I saw small groups of my cells all bunched up together—as though huddling for warmth, or from fear. Why they had done this is the great mystery of cancer. However, that image coupled with visions seen during sessions with ayahuasca convinced me that my cells had gotten out of line and were experiencing cellular disorientation. Moreover, I knew this situation wasn't caused by some invasive bacterium but by something from within.

My perception of what I needed to correct this cellular deformity and prevent its reoccurrence may be equally unscientific. My sense is that I needed to realign my cells and repair the electro-chemical communication system that links them together through the complex and poorly understood functions of DNA.

I can't explain how I have come to these conclusions. I have no background in science, and I am only beginning to study the fundamentals of the neurotransmitter systems, biochemistry, and entheogenic pharmacology. I am aware a little learning could prove to be a dangerous thing, as Alexander Pope once said. Nonetheless, I have formulated several rudimentary hypotheses, which I will attempt to explain.

My first hypothesis is that ayahuasca organically restores order and brings everything into realignment. In my experience, ayahuasca doesn't indiscriminately destroy cells, as chemotherapy does. Rather, ayahuasca serves to restore the normal, healthy alignment of cells while it seeks out and purges the aberrant ones that it finds while making its way throughout the body. It also seems to polish rough edges, illuminate dark corners, hone the senses, and—most importantly—ferret out physical (as well as psychic) detritus and purge it.

To use a mechanical model, it is comparable to fine-tuning an engine and changing the oil. That is basically how I see ayahuasca acting on me as it teaches my cells how not to get out of whack again.

Let me describe some of the experiences that have led me to these conclusions. About ten to fifteen minutes after ingestion, I typically begin to feel a force flickering throughout my body, growing in intensity to a ripple. Points of light flash intermittently as the energy force makes its rounds throughout my body. These flashes remind me of the little points of light that one sees in the optometrist's office when undergoing the test for peripheral vision (Visual Field Analyzer). As the minutes pass, this rippling sensation gets stronger, until they feel like Northern Lights surging in successive waves throughout my body.

In my experiences, this stage often continues for one to two hours before I begin to have any visions (I have been told this is a relatively long onset period). My subjective sense is that the vine is exploring every nook and cranny of my entire system, racing around to ensure that everything is in order. Any disorder it encounters is corrected, and all of the garbage is swept up to be carried to my visceral dumpster for eventual purging. Perhaps because I am in need of deep cleansing, this phase lasts longer for me than for most other people. With someone like myself who has had metastatic cancer, there is a lot of cleaning up to do.

Perhaps the most obvious aspect of ayahuasca work on the organic level is the purge. As with most others, ayahuasca makes me vomit. Unlike many others, however, I generally don't vomit until after my visions have faded, maybe four or more hours after ingestion. Again, I interpret the late vomiting similarly to the way I interpret the late onset of vision. The vine seems to need more time with me to do its cleanup work, gathering the detritus and bringing it to the trash bin. When the cleanup job is done, the vine presses the release button and the garbage gets dumped, or vomited, out. On two occasions, I have also experienced slight diarrhea, the other type of purging that *ayahuasqueros* report.

The purge seems to be the vine's way of eliminating physical as well as psychic toxins that don't belong inside a healthy body or mind. Although the act of purging is not pleasant, the remarkable cleansing effect can be felt immediately, and it often lingers for days or even weeks. I have come to view the purge as a rite of purification.

When the visions begin, they often seem to confirm my earlier sensations. Among the first things I see are the curling, spiraling, intertwining, self-propelled ribbons of varicolored transparent light, alternately taking on features of serpents and plants. Sometimes, they appear to be just ribbons of light. Inside each of them is a black double-helix skeleton that seems to propel it. Although the resemblance between these forms and the drawings of DNA that I have seen is stunning, I doubt that the images came from my memory. I saw the forms long before I read Jeremy Narby's book *The Cosmic Serpent* (1998) and began to associate the lights with DNA.

In any case, I have been impressed by the consistent reoccurrence of these ribbons during every ayahuasca experience, and I suspect that if one could see DNA in action, it would probably look much like what I have tried to describe. As the intensity and speed of the visions increase, the ribbons seem to well up from the deepest parts of my gut and the furthest reaches of my limbs, climbing, soaring, and bursting into brilliant showers of light, like enormous skyrockets. From time to time, I feel and see a powerful upswelling of a brilliant gold mass of energy, coming from deep within me, climaxing in an orgasmic burst into infinity. Following these surges of light, I feel I have undergone an internal cleansing, as though by some sort of cosmic Roto-Rooter.

I interpret these visions as manifestations of what the plant is doing inside me on the microscopic, organic level. The plant is doing its work, looking for dark corners to illuminate and malformations to correct, communicating with my cells through the chemical chain provided by our respective DNA. In plain words, the DNA of the vine is talking to mine. If, as Jeremy Narby and others have suggested, the DNA is the communication system of cells, then it may not be farfetched to suggest that the DNA of the plant could be talking to ours after it enters our electro-chemical systems and teaching our DNA about balance and alignment. In doing this, the plant could be serving to restore the symmetry that produces health and well-being.

To accept this interpretation of how ayahuasca works requires acceptance of the idea that plants can communicate, not only among themselves but with humans as well. We must accept the notion that, as my group leader once put it, "the plant knows what it is doing." Although the idea of the ayahuasca plant as teacher is probably as old as ayahuasca use itself, most Westerners—and scientists in particular—might find this idea preposterous because it suggests that the plant is intelligent, that it has a spirit, and that it can communicate. These are not easy concepts for Westerners to understand or accept. Yet, this is how I—a lifelong skeptic and pragmatist—now see the plant doing its work. And it has undeniably worked well for me.

Could this be pure fantasy on my part? Could it be that I have constructed from my imagination an account in order to explain my experiences? I don't think so. I have attempted to provide an accurate description of my experiences. I am convinced that my affair with the vine is largely responsible for my current state of good health.

The shamans of the Amazon have been using ayahuasca for healing purposes for centuries, during which they obviously have seen concrete results, not necessarily for curing cancer but certainly for treating a host of other diseases. As with other practitioners of folk medicine, they don't pursue modalities of treatment that don't work.

A considerable amount of anecdotal evidence suggests that ayahuasca does work in treating disease. However, most Westerners are locked into analytic mind-sets and, before they will believe, they need to see controlled studies on humans, with carefully measured data that can be scientifically evaluated. Such a study should not be difficult to conduct, if the obstacles of prohibition can be overcome. One way to do this is to conduct the study in a less repressive country. The other approach is to take on the DEA and challenge it to consider scientific inquiry into the world of entheogenic plants. It is my fervent hope that such studies will move forward in the near future.

There is much to be learned from the indigenous cultures that have worked with ayahuasca for many centuries—and from the plants themselves, if only we can learn how to tune in. I am eager to work more with people who not only respect and listen to the plant, but who also have learned how to interact with it in alternate realms. My hope is to learn some of that language myself, partly in order to help teach others to respect it. As a former professor, the teaching part should come easily. In my current role as a drug policy reformer, I am working to free this marvelous plant teacher from the structures that the DEA has so capriciously and arrogantly placed on it. I invite people who read this article to join me in this effort.

An Ethnobotanist's Dream

Glenn H. Shepard, Ph.D.

Ethnobotanist Glenn Shepard has spent years working with Machiguenga shamans in the Peruvian Amazon, and studying their knowledge about plants. Here, he describes a dream he had under the influence of a tobacco paste prepared by a shaman. Highly concentrated with banisteriopsis, *the powerful plant catalyst used in preparing ayahuasca brews, the Machiguenga tobacco paste takes Shepard on a fantastic journey to the future of Amazonian ethnobotany.*

IT WAS A BRILLIANT September afternoon at the end of the dry season in the Peruvian Amazon, when strong breezes and gathering clouds announce the coming of the long season of rains. I had walked an hour along a well-used path through the forest to the residence and gardens of Mariano and his family at Potsitakigia. Mariano, one of my key informants during many months of ethnographic and ethnobotanical research, was sitting in a rustic, open-sided construction thatched with palm leaves that was the unfinished kitchen area of his new house. We talked for a few minutes, and then he got a mischievous look in his eye, and said, "I've got something for you." He reached between the panels of palm thatch on the underside of the low roof and removed a short bamboo tube plugged with corn husks. He uncapped the tube and dug in with a pointed stick, extracting a few wads of sticky black substance. "What is that?" I asked. "*Opatsa seri,*" he replied. He put a pinch into his mouth and chewed, grimacing at the taste.

I was surprised. I had heard about *opatsa seri,* "tobacco paste," during some twelve prior months of fieldwork among the Matsigenka. Mariano and other storytellers had described this magical substance in legends about ancient times. *Opatsa seri,* a highly concentrated paste made of tobacco and *Banisteriopsis,* was the substance that first gave "Blowing Spirit," *Tasorintsi,* the transformative powers needed to create the world and all its creatures. It was also used by ancient shamans to change themselves into animals or fly to distant realms. But until that afternoon, none had hinted to me that this mythical substance was still manufactured and consumed. *Opatsa seri* was the philosopher's stone, the stuff of legend.

"Open your mouth," said Mariano, He removed the masticated black quid—about the size of a pencil eraser—from his own tongue and placed it on mine. "Chew."

The little piece of *opatsa seri* was perhaps the most bitter thing I had ever put in my mouth, tasting like a mixture of unsweetened coffee powder, coal tar and Vegemite. A dry, burning sensation slid down the back of my throat. "Is it bitter?" Mariano asked. "Very." I shook my head and winced. "Swallow," he said. I hiccupped a few times as the bitter quid descended, settling uneasily in my stomach.

Mariano explained the use of *opatsa seri* to me in this way. "You take *opatsa seri* in the afternoon. Not too late, or you won't be able to sleep, but like now, when the sun is over there [about 4 P.M.]. It makes you dream. Only good things. People, lots of people. Come back tomorrow and tell me if what I say is not true."

For the rest of the afternoon, I felt a mild and slightly queasy sense of stimulation, like drinking black coffee on an empty stomach. That night, my dreams were nothing short of fantastic. I had returned a decade in the future, and found the village transformed. Matsigenka ethnobotany had become the focus of international medical research. Doctors, chemists and botanists from around the world came and went from vast research facilities, fashioned as neo-Mayan pyramids of gleaming white stone. All the foreign visitors wore beautiful Matsigenka tunics decorated with geometric designs. Matsigenka had become a required language in medical schools around the world. I felt a sharp pang of jealousy when I met a team of Yankee doctors who spoke Matsigenka better than I, notwithstanding their distinct New York accent. I was given a tour of a labyrinthine museum of exquisite pre-Columbian artifacts and Matsigenka *objets d'art*. Then I was taken through endless rows of greenhouses and orchards, where hundreds of medicinal plants were being cultivated for cutting-edge medical research: aromatic herbs, fantastic fruit trees, beautiful flowers, succulent vines. Young Matsigenka botanists, fluent in English, explained the names and uses of different plants and showed me laboratories and clinics where researchers tested new drugs on human and animal subjects. The images were lucid and vivid, in full color, with clear sounds and smells. The dream seemed to last for many hours, and when I woke up it was dark. I wondered whether I had slept an entire day. But when I checked my watch, it was still very early in the morning: only a few hours had passed since I had fallen asleep. I took notes on the dream, amused by the more absurd parts but nonetheless intrigued by the powerful images, apparently induced by Mariano's "dream tobacco."

I went excitedly to Mariano's the next morning to tell him of my extraordinary dreams. He laughed, not surprised, and responded: "I told you so. Tobacco paste is *kepigari*, 'intoxicating.' It is very strong. It was calling to you, it wanted you. It took you to visit the *Saangariite,* the guardian spirits. They are very wise and good, like doctors and teachers. They can show you many things."

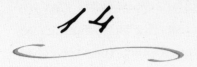

Shamans and Scientists

Jeremy Narby, Ph.D.

In 1999, three molecular biologists traveled to the Peruvian Amazon to see whether they could obtain biomolecular information in ceremonial ayahuasca sessions conducted by an indigenous shaman. Swiss-Canadian anthropologist Jeremy Narby reports on their experiences and the responses they received to their research questions. This unusual perspective on ethnopharmacology attest to the value of modern scientists and indigenous healers alike learning from the traditions of others.

THE MOLECULAR BIOLOGISTS had no previous experience of ayahuasca shamanism or of the Amazon, though they did have an interest in alternative healing traditions and shamanism. Their ages ranged from the late thirties to mid-sixties. One worked as a scientist in an American genomics company. Another was a professor at a French university and a member of the National Center for Scientific Research (CNRS). The third was a professor at a Swiss university and a director of research at a federal agriculture research station.

None of the scientists spoke Spanish, and the indigenous ayahuasquero did not speak English or French, so I translated for them. The first thing to report is that the scientists and the shaman had many long conversations. They did not cease to have things to say to one another. The shaman had been studying plants, as an ayahuasquero, for thirty-seven years. He answered the biologists's questions for days on end.

He also conducted nighttime ayahuasca sessions, in which the biologists took part. They saw many things in their visions, including DNA molecules and chromosomes.

The American biologist, who normally worked on deciphering the human genome, said she saw a chromosome from the perspective of a protein flying above a long strand of DNA. She saw DNA sequences known as "CpG islands," which she had been puzzling over at work, and which are found upstream of about sixty percent of all human genes. She saw they were structurally distinct from the surrounding DNA and that this structural difference allowed them to be easily accessed and therefore to serve as "landing pads" for transcription proteins, which dock on to the DNA molecule and make copies of precise genetic sequences. She said the idea that CpG island structure enables them to function as landing pads had not crossed her mind previously, and that genomic research would soon be able to verify this hypothesis.

The French professor had been studying the sperm duct of animals for many years, first in lizards, then in mice. When a sperm cell comes out of the testis and enters the sperm duct, it is incapable of fertilizing an egg. It only becomes fertile once it has traveled through the duct, where about fifty different kinds of proteins work on it. The professor and his team had spent years trying to understand which protein makes the sperm cell fertile. Understanding this could have implications for the development of a male contraceptive. He brought three questions to one of the ayahuasca sessions. First, was there a key protein that makes sperm cells fertile? Second, why had it not been possible to find the answer to that question after years of research? And, third, was the mouse the appropriate model for studying fertility in men?

He received answers from a voice that spoke in his visions. In reply to the first question, the voice said: "No, it is not a key protein. In this organ, there are no key proteins, just many different ones which have to act together for fertility to be achieved." To the second question, it said: "I already answered that with your first question." To the third question, it said: "This question is not important enough for me to answer. The answer can be found without ayahuasca. Try to work in another direction."

As for the Swiss professor, she had been working for years on modifying genes of tobacco and potato plants to protect them from viruses. Her intention was to produce plants that required less pesticides when grown on an industrial scale. Her work had been criticized by ecologists, who questioned the appropriateness of genetic engineering. She had taken their criticism to heart, and wanted to consult the shamanic sphere about whether it is appropriate to modify the tobacco genome to make the plant resistant to a virus. It so happens tobacco is an important plant in Amazonian shamanism. Shamans from many different indigenous societies say they speak in their visions with the "mother of tobacco," or the essence of the plant. The biologist reported that she spoke with the mother of tobacco during an ayahuasca-influenced meditation; this entity informed her that tobacco was pleased to serve people and all other species, including viruses. The mother of tobacco also informed the biologist that manipulating tobacco's genome was not a problem in itself, so long as it was done with the common good in mind. The biologist came away from this encounter with the understanding that genetic manipulations were best gauged case by case, in a way that takes into consideration the scientist's intention as well as the way in which the modified plants will be used by society.

In interviews conducted in their respective laboratories four months after the Amazonian experience, the three biologists agreed on a number of points. All three said the experience of ayahuasca shamanism changed their way of looking at themselves and at the world, as well as their appreciation of the capacities of the human mind. They all expressed great respect for the shaman's skill and knowledge. They all received information and advice about paths of research they were on. The two women reported contact with "plant teachers," which they experienced as independent entities; they both said that contacting a plant teacher had shifted their way of understanding reality. The man said that all the things he saw and learned in his visions were somehow already in his mind, but that ayahuasca had helped him see into his mind and put them together. He did not think he had experienced contact with an outside intelligence, but he did think ayahuasca was a powerful tool for exploring the mind.

The scientific information and imagery accessed in ayahuasca visions by the three biologists were certainly related to the information and images already in their minds. They did not have any big revelations. "Ayahuasca is not a shortcut to the Nobel prize," the French professor remarked. They all said that ayahuasca shamanism was a harder path to knowledge than science, and as scientists, they found specific difficulties with it. For example, getting knowledge from an ayahuasca experience involves a highly emotional, subjective experience that is not reproducible. One cannot have the same ayahuasca experience twice, nor can somebody else have the same ayahuasca experience as oneself. This makes it almost contrary to the method of science, which consists of designing objective experiments that can be repeated by anyone, anywhere, anytime.

The scientists said that more research was needed; and that this would require preparing questions carefully, and working with qualified shamans in well-defined conditions. And they are all planning to return to the Amazon at some point to continue working on this.

They conducted this preliminary experiment over two weeks. Afterward, they visited a school for bilingual, intercultural education, where young women and men from fourteen indigenous societies are learning to teach indigenous knowledge and science, in their mother tongue and in Spanish. They are Aguaruna, Shipibo, Huitoto, Ashaninca and so on. The school's goal is to train indigenous primary school teachers. Each people has elected an old "indigenous specialist" to work at the school as the keeper and teacher of its knowledge, language and lore.

The scientists met with the school's director and with the old indigenous specialists. They spoke positively about their recent experience with an indigenous shaman. But several of the specialists warned them about the abuses that can occur with ayahuasca shamanism. They said that sorcerers worked with ayahuasca and shot darts into people to cause disease. They said ayahuasca was double-edged. "The plant can show you things that will harm you," said one. They emphasized that using ayahuasca required the presence of a well-trained and talented ayahuasquero.

The specialists asked the scientists about science: What was its nature? Where did its center lie? One of the scientists replied that science was fragmented into many disciplines and was practiced in many countries. He went on to say that he thought it was very important that young indigenous people learned about science, because it was currently the dominant form of knowledge around the world. In reply, one specialist said he thought this was true, but he also thought that the scientists might consider sending their children to the Amazon to learn about indigenous knowledge. That way, he said, they, too, would benefit from a complete education.

Once everybody had spoken, the Aguaruna director of the school thanked us for our visit and said: "Here in the Amazon, our knowledge has been taken many times by others, but we have never received any benefits from it. Now we would like to see some returns." He said that an agreement regarding the compensation of indigenous knowledge should be established before any further research was conducted.

This experiment seemed to show that scientists can learn things by working with indigenous Amazonian shamans.

Some observers have suggested that shamanism, as classically defined, is reaching its end. But bringing shamans and scientists together seems more like a beginning.

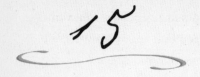

Ritual Approaches to Working with Sacred Medicine Plants

An Interview with Ralph Metzner, Ph.D.

One of the most productive pioneer investigators of hallucinogens over the last several decades has been psychologist Ralph Metzner. A protégé of Timothy Leary and Richard Alpert while a graduate student at Harvard in the early 1960s, Dr. Metzner has been a prolific chronicler of the evolving relationship between hallucinogens and society. Going beyond Leary's emphasis of set and setting, Metzner has elaborated on the value of shamanic structures to optimizing outcome and minimizing risk. In this interview with Timothy White, Metzner shares many of his insights on traditional and contemporary models of hallucinogen use.

TIMOTHY WHITE: *You are known as a leading authority on the subjects of psychedelic mysticism, altered states of consciousness, and ecospiritual philosophy. How did you develop those interests?*

RALPH METZNER: As a psychologist, I have been involved in studying human consciousness—including psychedelic states—for over thirty-five years. My first psychedelic experience was in 1961 when I was a graduate student at Harvard. For several years, I worked with Timothy Leary and Richard Alpert, doing research on potential therapeutic and creative applications of psychedelics, particularly LSD and psilocybin.

In the late 1960s, I stopped taking psychedelics, for both political and health reasons, and I shifted my studies to exploring non-drug methods for transforming consciousness. I got involved in various Eastern and Western esoteric traditions, including *hatha yoga,* meditation, and alchemy. I also worked with several experimental forms of psychotherapy involving body work, breath work, and deep trance states.

In the late 1970s, I moved back to San Francisco where I was the academic dean for ten years at the California Institute of Integral Studies. While at CIIS, I was introduced to the work of Michael Harner, who was teaching the use of drumming, or auditory driving, to induce non-ordinary states of consciousness. I resonated with several aspects of Harner's approach: setting a clear purpose for the journey, paying attention to going into alternate realities and coming back, and using the journey to bring back practical solutions to problems. A secondary advantage of his approach was that one could conduct many drumming journeys in a day, which I thought could prove useful for psychotherapeutic applications. That work sparked my interest in experiential shamanism.

For a time, I explored a variety of Native American practices, including fasting, wilderness vision questing, and sweat lodge ceremonies. Simultaneously, I began to read the work of Weston LaBarre, Richard Evans Schultes, Peter Furst, and others who had been documenting shamanic methods of working with psychoactive plants. As a clinical psychologist, I had somehow overlooked the wealth of information in the anthropological literature on the indigenous use of sacred plants.

I was intrigued to learn that certain psychedelic plants, such as peyote and ayahuasca, have been used safely in indigenous traditions for hundreds, if not thousands, of years. One reason that I had stopped using synthetic psychedelics was possible safety issues surrounding the unknown long-term effects of these drugs.

WHITE: *I sometimes like to preach that the true art of shamanism is not* *about tripping out into other realms but about bringing the healing insights and energies of those realms back into this world—it's about manifesting Heaven on Earth.*

I understand that you have worked with a considerable variety of plant sacraments—including peyote, San Pedro, psilocybin mushrooms, and ayahuasca—in both traditional shamanic rituals and more contemporary ceremonial contexts. Could you provide some insights into how different ceremonial formats influence the entheogenic experience?

METZNER: Actually, I have only limited experience working with medicine plants within indigenous shamanic ceremonies. I have participated in a few Native American Church ceremonies. My experiences working with *iboga* (the source of ibogaine), San Pedro, and mushrooms have been almost entirely within neoshamanic and psychotherapeutic contexts. My most extensive field research has been focused on studying the ayahuasca traditions in South America, partly because the religious use of ayahuasca has been legal in Brazil and partly because they offer a variety of different ritual approaches to the same psychedelic.

In the Amazon, ayahuasca has been used in indigenous shamanic ceremonies for centuries. Although these ayahuasca ceremonies vary slightly from tribe to tribe, many of them have similar ritual elements. During the twentieth century, the traditional ayahuasca rituals were adapted and transformed by acculturated Indians and mestizos into a variety of individualized yet culturally similar ceremonies. Most of these mestizo ceremonies follow basic shamanic ceremonial patterns: specially trained shamans or healers, known as *ayahuasqueros,* and their clients consume ayahuasca, and then the healers spend the night singing special ayahuasca songs, known as *icaros,* which are used to communicate with spirit powers for healing or divination.

As a result of my interest in ayahuasca shamanism, I learned that, in addition to the indigenous and mestizo ayahuasca ceremonies, there were three interesting new folk religions in Brazil—the Santo Daime, Uniao de Vegetal (UDV), and Barquinia—that all use ayahuasca, also known as *daime* and *hoasca,* as the main sacrament in communal ceremonies. Each

of these folk religions was founded by a rubber tapper who was first introduced to the use of ayahuasca by mestizo and Indian healers. Although
two of these churches were founded fairly recently—in the 1950s—each
of them already has thousands of members in Brazil. Two of the churches
have even established satellite centers in Europe and North America.

When I began to hear reports that many of the participants involved in the
ayahuasca churches were experiencing profound spiritual transformations
as a result of their experiences with the ayahuasca, I was intrigued. The
Brazilian government had legalized the religious use of ayahuasca after it conducted an extensive scientific and sociological study of the three traditions.

WHITE: *Would you talk about your experiences at the Santo Daime ceremonies and what you learned?*

METZNER: Santo Daime is a highly syncretic tradition, combining
Christian, spiritualistic, and psychotherapeutic elements. The Santo Daime
Church (as well as the other groups) has brought the use of ayahuasca out
of the context of small shamanic healing rituals and has greatly expanded
its use by making this profoundly transformative spiritual experience available to a large number and wide spectrum of people.

If you define shamanism as an ecstatic journey by a shaman into alternate realms for healing or divination, then the ayahuasca churches don't
practice pure forms of shamanism. In my observation, the intent of the
Daime ceremony seems to be aimed at generating communal mystical experiences, as opposed to individual visions. In Daime, the traditional shamans
have been replaced by priests and officials, and the focus of the ceremonies
has shifted away from the dramatic shamanic healings to encouraging self-
healing and strengthening community bonds.

In certain respects, the Daime ceremonies remind me of a combination
of the Native American Church peyote meeting and old-time gospel meeting. The participants all take standardized doses of the Daime sacrament
and then stay up all night long, singing special songs throughout the night.
Unlike the Native American Church, the Daime ceremonies include a lot
of dancing and swaying, which is reminiscent of gospel meetings.

Some people have difficulty relating to the structure of the Santo Daime ceremony and its emphasis on Judeo-Christian religious motifs. Daime songs frequently invoke Jesus, Mary, and Old Testament figures such as Solomon, but they also invoke their own deities. There are also hymns to invoke the spirits of their two sacred plant medicines—the Daime and Santa Maria (cannabis)—and they have other songs to invoke the sun, the moon, and the stars, as well as the spirit of the forest. Many Daime songs also speak of letting go of envy, anger, and bad feelings, as well as bringing in love.

One thing I like about the Daime ceremonies is that they involve very little talking. They have certain prayers, such as the Lord's Prayer, which is recited at the opening and close of the ceremony. But during the ceremony itself, there is just a lot of singing and dancing.

In Daime, they do this dance where everyone is dancing in two semicircles, with the men on one side and the women on the other. You move two steps to the left and then two steps to the right. The movements are synchronized, creating a wave that carries you along. The dance becomes almost effortless, and you can dance that way for six to eight hours, which is done. If you were dancing by yourself, you couldn't do it for very long at all.

Some Daime people—individuals who have been doing sessions for many years—have told me that they sometimes experience the same ceremony taking place on the astral plane, and they are able to consciously participate in both ceremonies simultaneously. They say that the Daime songs have all been brought through, or channeled, from the astral plane and that these songs interact with or activate the medicine in ways which allow practitioners to work multidimensionally during the ceremonies.

Wherever the songs came from, they enhance the experience. During one Daime session I attended in Brazil, I felt this wave of empathic energy flowing through one particular song. I felt it move first through the whole group and then it extended into the larger community. Then, it extended to embrace the whole Amazonian rainforest, the whole planet, the entire solar system, and even beyond. When it was almost over, the song brought the energy back down to where we were—in the present. It had opened all these other levels of spiritual awareness, and it brought the awareness of those other dimensions into the physical realms.

The Daime songs also have a rhythmic quality that seems to carry one along. At one Daime session, I took a standard dose, but it turned out to be too intense for me. I couldn't stand up; I had to lie down. I saw myself in a past life scene in the middle of a battlefield, covered in blood and gore. I was very glad that the others kept singing and dancing right next to me, because it helped me go through that vision. If I had been by myself, it might have been really hard. They kept the song going, and after ten or fifteen minutes, everything was okay.

I have a lot of respect for the Daime ceremony. If you are going to do ayahuasca in large groups of twenty, forty, or a hundred people, then that is the way to do it. The ritual provides a structure that supports personal healing and also keeps people from infringing upon each other.

In the 1980s, I spent a lot of time pondering why Westerners had been so quick to abuse and misuse psychoactives, whereas Native Americans had successfully integrated the religious use of peyote into many of their cultures in a relatively short time. I concluded that the primary difference was that Native Americans used peyote within communal ceremonies that simultaneously encouraged religious, medicinal, and psychotherapeutic purposes. The ceremonies resulted in experiences that were much more meaningful than the average psychedelic trip.

When I began studying shamanic healing and divination ceremonies, I noticed that most shamanic ceremonies—particularly those that used psychedelics—were carefully structured experiences. I could see that the ceremonies provided both a meaningful focus and a safe container for the psychedelic experience.

I noticed parallels between elements of the ceremonial structures and Leary's now famous "set and setting" hypothesis. His theory was that psychedelics function as catalysts or amplifiers, and that the content of a psychedelic experience is a function of the *set* (the person's intention, expectations, and basic personality) and the *setting* (the immediate physical and social environment). In short, psychedelics may shift a person into altered states of consciousness, but the content of those states depends largely upon the intentions and expectations of the user.

WHITE: *I basically agree with Leary's theory of set and setting, and I understand that he was trying to show that psychedelics were different from, and couldn't be administered in the same way as, most pharmaceutical medicines. However, I believe that we must also consider the signature, or characteristic traits, of the psychedelic used. In my experience, peyote typically catalyzes a very different experience than, for example, psilocybin mushrooms or LSD. Peyote tends to generate heartfelt feelings of love and unity, whereas LSD has always impressed me as emotionally detached and very mental.*

METZNER: I, too, have noticed that there are some qualitative differences between how one experiences different medicines in one's spirit, mind, and body. For instance, psilocybin mushrooms seem to produce a pure nervous system response. The Mazatecs speak of the mushrooms giving birth to language. The mushroom spirits seem to be elf-like beings or little children—as Mazatec shaman Maria Sabina called them—who like to laugh and play. They seem to exhibit a brilliant, scintillating, and tricksterish humor, and they seem benevolent, very sweet, and very magical.

Ayahuasca has some of those qualities, too, but it also has a gut-wrenching nature. Its spirits tend to be serpentine—the serpents of the air, water, the earth, the fire. Jeremy Narby argues in his book, *The Cosmic Serpent,* that the serpentine visions associated with ayahuasca basically derive from a shamanic awareness of the DNA molecule, which the mind interprets as serpent spirits.

Considering that *iboga* is traditionally used by the Fang tribe of Africa in order to interact with ancestors, I find it interesting that ibogaine has become the preferred psychedelic medicine of many psychotherapists. It may be that the ibogaine stimulates early memories, which would make it useful in psychoanalytic work focused on parental issues. However, it may also be that its reputation for contacting ancestors appeals to the imagination of psychotherapists.

Some of the qualitative differences between plant psychedelics may be due to their different pharmacological properties. However, they may also reflect the different cultural and personal expectations of the individual.

WHITE: *When I first began working with psychedelics in college, I assumed that the differences between medicine plants were probably due to*

their pharmacological constituents. Over the years of working with plant sacra-
ments, I have noticed that the signature traits of a plant medicine can't always
be explained by the plant's pharmacological makeup.

Take the example of the San Pedro cactus and peyote. The first time I took
San Pedro, at a ceremony in 1985 led by the Peruvian shaman don Eduardo
Calderon, I was expecting a peyote-like experience. Everything I had read
about San Pedro had indicated that, pharmacologically, it is very similar to
peyote. I was very surprised to find that it had a totally different feel for me.
The San Pedro engendered some of the same empathic quality as peyote, but
its overall energy was much more diffused.

In certain respects, the San Pedro reminded me of mushrooms. Although it
didn't produce the vivid visions that are typical of mushrooms, I experienced
a kind of diffusive moon energy that I associate with mushrooms. The next
day, when I spoke to don Eduardo about my experience, he reminded me that
San Pedro is a moon plant—it blossoms under the moon. In contrast, peyote
seems to contain a lot of solar energy, which fits the fact that it grows in high,
sunny deserts.

METZNER: You may be right. I have worked with both San Pedro
cactus and peyote, as well as mescaline's closest synthetic equivalent,
MDMA, and I have noticed that each has a slightly different feel. In my
experience, San Pedro can engender a certain heartfulness and an emotional awareness similar to a peyote experience, but it also tends to produce a more individual, meditative experience, particularly when taken in
low dosages.

If there are differences, they may be due to the way that the plants grow.
The San Pedro cactus has this immense growing power. People often comment that San Pedro produces an expansive feeling inside them. In comparison, peyote plants grow very slowly and stay close to the ground. Peyote
tends to produce a very focused and grounded experience. However, I
would suggest that the differences you experienced may also have been
influenced by the ceremonial contexts in which the plant medicines were
taken.

When I first started conducting research on ayahuasca groups, I was
aware that ayahuasca is used in some Amazonian societies to teach people

about their environment. I wondered what would happen when people started taking ayahuasca in Europe and North America. Would the medicine teach northern peoples about the Amazonian rainforest? I have found that some people do get rainforest imagery and find themselves in the rainforests with jaguars and snakes. Some people find themselves relating to their local environments, and some end up exploring their own psyches.

WHITE: *Ceremonial contexts undoubtedly influence the psychedelic experience, but I have also noticed that when different plant medicines are used with the same structures, they can still generate different experiences. For instance, during the late 1970s, I worked with a ceremonial leader who used to lead medicine circles using a mix of peyote and psilocybin mushrooms. Several times when he had difficulty obtaining peyote, he conducted the ceremony using only mushrooms. I noticed that the mushrooms seemed to catalyze a broad variety of emotional experiences, ranging from deep cathartic processing to uncontrolled laughter—sometimes within the same ceremony. In contrast, peyote by itself always seems to produce a much more cohesive, communal empathic experience.*

METZNER: There are obvious differences between the feel and intensity of different medicine plants. However, my experiences working with various medicines suggest that the individual's intention influences the content of psychedelic experience as much, or even more, than the pharmacological properties of the medicine. If someone sets the intention of obtaining shamanic knowledge—for healing, prophecy, or survival then that's usually what they get, regardless of what medicine plants they happen to take. If people focus on working out things from their childhood, then they tend to see images that relate to their childhood. If they focus on spiritual transformation or understanding the universe, then the psychedelic tends to reveal spiritual insights or knowledge. I think that's why many entheogenic rituals often begin by setting the focus or intent of the ceremony.

WHITE: *I agree that it is most useful to set one's intent or purpose when working with medicines. However, I must add that the spirits of medicine plants have wills of their own and may override our conscious intentions.*

They have a tendency to say, "You were looking for something you wanted, but I'm going to show you what you really need to see."

METZNER: Psilocybin mushrooms are great at doing that sort of thing. They might say, "You want to know about your relationship with your father. Take a look at this galactic perspective."

I had an interesting experience along that line when I started working with *iboga*. I was really connecting with the medicine. I saw African village scenes with women dancing and singing and children playing. Then, all of a sudden, I saw a little, white-skinned child wearing European clothing. I remember thinking, "What's he doing here?" He didn't seem to belong in the vision. I decided it was a personal memory image from my childhood.

Then I was shown a whole series of images or visions that gave me psychological insight into my relationship with my mother. The images were like little vignettes, or extracts, from a movie of my life. This offered me a gestalt of my relationship with my mother, but it was essentially a psychological experience.

Then, after a while, I was back in the African environment with people dancing. A male figure came towards me and stood in front of me. I couldn't see his face because he had a hat on, but I could see his hands and feet. He was almost an Odin type of character, but he was wearing shorts. He was making these strange hand gestures towards me that led me to understand he had been showing me the images in my mind. I realized that he was the spirit of the *iboga* and he was teaching me about my psychological history. I was blown away. I never expected to experience anything like that.

It is not uncommon for people taking psychedelics to perceive or feel the presence of deities or spirits from other cultures, including some with whom they have no genetic, biographical, or cultural connection. While working on my most recent book, I interviewed some people in European ayahuasca groups who had had visions of Egyptian gods and goddesses, and some came up with details beyond their conscious knowledge. In one case, they didn't even recognize that the images were Egyptian. These cases could involve some type of past life memory.

Once when I was taking mushrooms—which I have always associated with Mesoamerican shamanism—I had a vision of myself sitting in a Shiva posture in a Shiva temple. I've had other visions along that line, which make me think that I may have had past lives in India as a Shiva devotee.

WHITE: *I have noticed that the shamanic use of images—such as climbing up a tree or going down a hole—seems to function as a mental focusing device that may allow us to seek and find certain information on the cosmic internet. It is useful to set clear parameters or coordinates when we are searching through the limitless realms of alternate realities.*

METZNER: Yes, I think that is also why shamans often employ crystals, feathers, or other ceremonial paraphernalia. They function as visualization aids for focusing imaginal processes, but there is also more to shamanic process than that. In most shamanic traditions, there are usually designated steps that the shaman goes through in divination rituals. You go there, you do this, you make this sound, you think this thought.

Based on Leary's axiom that set and setting determine the content and nature of psychedelic experiences, it seemed to me that shamanic rituals could be seen as structures of set and setting that had been found to enhance healing and divination work. On the assumption that the most common ritual elements were the most important, I decided to start by identifying those ritual elements that appeared in many, if not most, shamanic ceremonies. Then I tried to understand how those elements might support the purpose of healing and divination.

Let me briefly identify some key ritual elements that can be found in well-known entheogenic healing ceremonies. I have already described how in the Daime rituals, participants take mild doses of the sacrament. Then they dance in circles around a central altar table, and they sing special songs throughout the night. Similar elements are found in many other ceremonies.

In the all-night peyote ceremonies of the Native American Church, participants sit in a circle on the ground around a blazing fire. The ceremony is led by a roadman, who is helped by several assistants. After consuming peyote in several forms, participants take turns singing special peyote songs to the accompaniment of a rattle and the rapid, rhythmic beat of a waterdrum.

In the South American Andes, healers and patients drink extracts of the San Pedro cactus in rituals held at night, usually sitting in front of a *mesa,* or altar, covered with symbolic figurines and objects, but sometimes around a fire. The *curandero,* or healer, chants for extended periods and occasionally leads the participants in ritual actions.

In the mushroom *veladas* of the Mazatecs, most of the ritual is conducted in the dark, but it is still focused around an altar containing candles and images. The healer, who is often a woman, continues to chant poetic songs throughout most of the night.

In the Bwiti cult practiced by the Fang people in Gabon, Africa, initiates drink the psychedelic plant *iboga,* and they are then guided through a powerful death-rebirth experience that allows them to speak with ancestor spirits. Initiates sit on the floor in a temple, focused on an altar with images of deities and ancestors. There is much chanting and drumming, as well as some dancing during the all-night ceremony.

Based on descriptions found in anthropological literature, I found it fairly easy to come up with a list of common ritual elements—the tendency to hold ceremonies at night, the use of moderate dosages of psychedelics, the ritual format of circles, the presence of a ceremonial leader, and the prolonged use of rhythmic drumming, singing, or dancing. However, it was only after I began to participate in a variety of entheogenic ceremonies that I began to fully appreciate how these elements contribute to the healing and divinatory processes.

One of the most prevalent ritual elements is that shamanic healings are generally conducted at night, in complete darkness or low light. Although it may be tempting to assume indigenous cultures hold their ceremonies at night for practical reasons, such as not to interfere with daytime activities, I think the primary reason is that darkness and low light conditions tend to facilitate the emergence of visions.

Visions play a key role in many shamanic traditions. We already know that the classical shamanic healings of Siberia typically involved some form of visionary journey during which the shaman contacts spirits or deities in alternate realities and endeavors to bring back hidden knowledge from the spirit worlds.

In most New World entheogenic healing traditions, shamans say that they receive hidden knowledge directly from the sacred plants, which are referred to either as deities or as "plant teachers." It is said that there is a spirit intelligence associated with the plants, and that the spirit communicates with those who ingest the medicine. Since ingesting plant medicines and conducting ceremonies in the dark both seem to help facilitate visions, I concluded that nighttime visions play a key role in shamanic healings, as well as divinatory sessions.

My second observation was that shamanic chanting or singing seemed to be essential to the success of the healing or divinatory process. In many cultures, the role of the shaman, *curandero,* or healer is usually considered essential to the healing process. Since in most traditional entheogenic rituals, the shaman does all or much of the singing, I originally thought that the verbal messages of the songs might help reprogram the consciousness of the patients or participants. I could see that the poetic chants of the Mazatec shamans and the elaborate hymns of the Daime might serve a similar transformative function.

However, in many shamanic traditions, the ceremonial songs have very simple, standardized lyrics, and some only use phonemes or nonsense syllables, so I kept looking. Then I noticed that the chants used in entheogenic rituals tend to have a fairly rapid rhythm, and they are often accompanied by rhythmic rattling or drumming. Since the pulse of these songs is often similar to the rhythmic beat used in shamanic drumming journeys, I came to think that the primary function of the rhythmic chanting might be to provide support for keeping the flow of visions moving.

WHITE: *You also mentioned the ritual use of circles and the presence of ceremonial leaders as being important ritual elements. How do they enhance the healing and divinatory processes?*

METZNER: In most traditional shamanic ceremonies, the shaman or healer plays a dominant role. The other participants usually sit in a circle or semicircle around either the shaman or a central altar. At a practical level, the circle format allows the participants to see what the shaman is doing, and the shaman to keep watch over everyone. However, there is another, more fundamental reason the circle structures.

The circle is a very ancient and natural structure for bringing people together in a cooperative manner. As far back as we know, people have gotten together to sit in circles around a fire, telling stories of their journeys and adventures, both inner and outer. I think that there is something inherently supportive and healing about doing rituals in circle formats.

The inherent healing power of gathering in ritual circles can be seen clearly in the group work referred to as Councils or Wisdom Circles. Although no psychoactives are used in these councils, their simple ritual format often inspires profound spiritual experiences. A key part of the council process is that people sit in a circle, and they pass a talking-staff around, taking turns speaking or singing. The person who is holding the staff has the floor, and the others listen to him or her with complete respect and attention. Everyone gets their say, and there is no debate or questioning.

Over the past decade, I have been watching the growth in Europe and the U.S. of some new psychedelic movements, ranging from popular *raves,* where young people take psychoactives such as ecstasy and then dance all night to loud music, to new psychotherapeutic groups, which may incorporate an eclectic mix of spiritual, shamanic, and psychotherapeutic approaches. Because of my interest in shamanism, I have been particularly interested in the development of some neoshamanic medicine groups that use psychedelics within shamanistic formats for personal healing and spiritual growth.

Several of these neoshamanic medicine groups utilize ceremonies similar to the Council circles. The participants typically consume some form of sacred plant medicine and then they spend the night passing a staff around a circle, taking turns singing or expressing themselves. Although these ceremonies tend to be less formal than the Native American Church and the Brazilian *hoasca* folk religions, they are definitely religious or spiritual in nature.

Many of the participants in these groups are interested in spiritual development, and many have studied other spiritual practices, such as Buddhist *vipassana* meditations, tantra yoga, and holotropic breathwork. Most of the participants are also well educated about psychedelics and they understand the importance of set and setting, so they have developed alternatives to fixed rituals. Often, the participants start each session by shar-ing their intentions and goals, which can vary from spiritual growth to psy-chotherapeutic healing to connecting with shamanic allies.

WHITE: *You mentioned that the use of moderate doses of psychedelics was a common cross-cultural feature of entheogenic ceremonies. That may be the case in Daime ceremonies, but in many traditional ayahuasca ceremonies, the shamans often take fairly strong dosages.*

METZNER: In the traditional ayahuasca ceremonies, shamans some-times take as much as their patients, or even more. However, those sha-mans have usually undergone extended training, developing their control so that they don't lose themselves in visions.

When powerful psychedelics, such as ayahuasca or mushrooms, are used in ceremonies, individuals occasionally get in touch with very deep emotional issues. In those ayahuasca ceremonies where strong doses are used, one hears a lot of heaving and sobbing, groaning and moaning.

I have noticed that the doses given out at most Daime ceremonies are not usually as strong as those used in traditional ayahuasca ceremonies. The standardized doses in Daime seem to be calculated to take one to the edge without pushing one over. If I closed my eyes, I might see visions, but if I opened my eyes, I would see the community. When there may be fifty to a hundred participants dancing in circles, and the movements are very synchronized, it is vital for everyone to stay reasonably focused.

Daime practitioners say that they take just enough ayahuasca to mag-nify the inner dimensions—the emotional or astral body, the mental body, and so on. Then they use the group singing and dancing to build a com-munal consciousness that goes beyond the personal. Part of the Daime practice involves developing that connection and becoming comfortable with that transpersonal link.

During the early research on psychotherapeutic uses of psychedelics, participants were purposefully given strong psychedelic dosages in order to help them get in touch with very deep issues. The problem is that when powerful psychedelics like LSD or psilocybin mushrooms are used, indi-viduals may get in touch with very deep emotional issues and regress into pre-rational states. For safety reasons, the leaders and assistants in these psychotherapy groups often stayed sober in order to function as designated helpers for the sessions.

In the early days of psychedelic therapy, it was almost unthinkable for the therapist to take the substance with the patient. However, Leary and others realized that it was essential that the therapist was personally familiar with the psychedelic being used, so he or she could understand and relate to what the patients were going through. It was generally found that when therapists took psilocybin with the other participants they could sometimes relate better, but they had problems staying focused on working therapeutically with the patients.

In some neoshamanic medicine groups, the leaders and assistants may take small amounts of the psychedelic in order to help them tune in to participants. However, they seldom take much, because they may be needed to provide damage control at the time-space level, helping make sure that participants don't disturb each other or do something dangerous, such as knock over a candle and start a fire.

WHITE: *Usually, when someone is having a hard time in a shamanic ceremony, the shaman may perform some form of shamanic intervention, such as incensing the individual or doing feather work, which takes care of the problem. Have you ever observed that sort of shamanic intervention in the neoshamanic groups that you have observed?*

METZNER: Most Westerners don't usually intervene in the same ways that a traditional shaman might, because they haven't gone through shamanic training. In some neoshamanic medicine circles that I have visited, I have occasionally seen some forms of shamanic intervention when people are not feeling well. For instance, the leader may use mantras or guided visualizations to help people find their way back to their center when they get lost.

In some neoshamanic circles, the role of the ceremonial leader tends to be downplayed and many of the leadership functions have been transferred to the cooperative circle participants. I have seen participants in these groups send healing energy—through chanting or direct energy channeling—to individuals having trouble.

In these medicine circles, participants usually take moderate dosages of the psychedelic, enough to enhance their visions without losing their focus through the night. Even with only moderate dosages, it takes considerable discipline and focus to stay present in the circle, sing, and remember the structure. Participants seldom lose total control, but occasionally individuals have difficulty actively participating in the circle. Some groups handle such situations by announcing in advance that it is okay not to sing, that people can just pass the staff to the next person if they don't feel up to singing. There is no judgment about that.

Occasionally, I have seen leaders and assistants resort to physical intervention when individuals lost control and started disturbing others in the circle. One time, I observed a medicine circle where two people who had taken a lot of LSD couldn't stop talking. When some of the others in the circle reminded them that they had made an agreement to respect the circle rules, they agreed to stop talking, but they still couldn't stop babbling. Their babbling was distracting and disturbing the others. Eventually, several assistants intervened and attempted to move them to another room, but then the two totally freaked out.

Later, the two said they had panicked when the attempt was made to move them out of the circle. They regarded the circle as their life raft, and they didn't want to be moved. They weren't able to take the staff and sit up and sing, but they felt safer being able to lie there. The circle seems to provide a container or safety net for people who can't keep it together.

WHITE: *In the Native American Church, there is a useful rule that if you take the medicine, you should stay in the ceremony, so that the leader can watch over and take care of you. They don't want people taking the medicine and then wandering around outside the safety of ceremony.*

METZNER: The Santo Daime and UDV churches in Brazil have similar rules. Of course, some Americans don't like any rules; they want to be free to do as they please.

My suggestion is that if people don't like the rules and style of a particular church, they shouldn't go to that church. One wouldn't walk into a Protestant or Catholic church and insist on being free to do whatever one wants.

WHITE: *I think it may actually be prudent to restrict the use of the more powerful psychedelics to certain types of controlled situations, such as psycho-*

therapy groups, religious ceremonies, or special retreat centers. One of the lessons that I hope we learned during the sixties was that unbridled access to psyche-delics did lead to occasional abuses, such as the spiking of punch at parties.

METZNER: Even during the early 1960s, such practices were never condoned by the psychotherapy community. Leary was very adamant that one must never give consciousness-altering substances to someone without his or her knowledge and permission.

Responsibility is the key issue. One doesn't see that sort of problem around the *hoasca* churches or the Native American Church, where psychedelics are used respectfully and responsibly.

WHITE: *Do you think there is any chance that the United States or other countries will follow the example of Brazil and adopt a more tolerant attitude toward the religious use of psychedelics?*

METZNER: The issues surrounding the legalization of psychoactives are very complicated—and frequently very irrational. One of the problems in the United States is that psychedelics have been mistakenly lumped together with the addictive drugs—heroin, cocaine, and crack. I think it is vital to distinguish between the consciousness-contracting, antisocial nature of addictive drugs and the consciousness-expanding, psychotherapeutic nature of psychedelics and hallucinogens.

WHITE: *In my opinion, there is no justification for putting natural medicine plants on the federal controlled substance lists, particularly when there is ample evidence that peyote, San Pedro, and ayahuasca are nonaddictive, physically benign, and socially benevolent.*

There is considerable historical evidence that peyote was originally banned because it competed with the efforts of missionaries who wanted to Christianize Native Americans. At the turn of this century, Indian agents and missionaries would lie in wait for peyote ceremonies. They would confiscate the peyote, destroy the tipis and sacred medicine objects, and throw participants into jail, allegedly for intoxication.

METZNER: I personally think that the wholesale prohibitions against psychoactives and psychedelics are a holdover from our culture's puritanical past. The religious right still views psychoactives as recreational diversions that will lead a person into a life of crime, sin, and self-destruction.

By now, it is absolutely clear that marijuana doesn't turn people into raving maniacs or dope fiends, yet there are people who continue to oppose the legalization of its medical use. It is revealing that the most frequent objection to legalizing the medical use of marijuana is that it might result in its use by some recreationalists.

There is no inherent reason why society can't distinguish between the medical use of a substance and its recreational use. We allow doctors to prescribe the use of some highly addictive drugs—including morphine and codeine.

We should also be able to distinguish between the sacramental use of a plant and its recreational use. During the great alcohol prohibition, the government distinguished between the sacramental use of wine in Christian communion rites and the recreational use of wine.

We should be able to keep the issues separate, and we should restrict only the abuse—not the use—of psychoactives. The irony is that we have legalized the recreational use of alcohol, and alcohol abuse is infinitely more dangerous and socially destructive than marijuana and many plant psychedelics.

By now, it should be clear that prohibitions seldom work. They do little beyond lining the pockets of organized crime and creating a need for more jails; they certainly don't discourage usage. The primary reason people repealed the Eighteenth Amendment that had banned the sale of alcohol was that it created more problems than it solved.

We have had marijuana prohibition for sixty years, and it certainly hasn't stopped people from using marijuana. In countries with prohibitions—like the U.S. and Ireland—usage among teenagers is currently somewhere around twenty-five percent. In contrast, only nine or ten percent of Dutch teenagers use marijuana, and it has been legally available in Holland now for twenty years.

Europeans are years ahead of Americans in these areas. There is considerable legitimate research being done in Europe on medical and psychotherapeutic applications of psychedelics. The Dutch have launched several biomedical research projects aimed at testing medicinal and psychotherapeutic uses of ibogaine and ayahuasca. One project has already shown ayahuasca to be an effective psychotherapeutic treatment for alcoholism and drug addiction, partly because it has a very strong purging effect and partly because it changes consciousness. I predict that psychotherapeutic use of ayahuasca will be legalized in Europe fairly soon.

I think that some medical and psychotherapeutic uses of psychedelics may be legalized in this country within the not-too-distant future. A small number of research projects exploring potential medical applications of psychedelics have already been approved by the Drug Enforcement Agency. Ibogaine is currently being tested as a treatment for countering cocaine addiction. MDMA is being investigated for the amelioration of pain and stress in terminal cancer patients.

WHITE: *I wish I could be as optimistic as you. However, the U.S. government has shown that it is irrationally resistant to legalizing the religious use of psychedelics. Every scientific study that has been conducted on peyote has shown that it is a benign, nonaddictive plant medicine, and anthropologists have been documenting the benevolent nature of peyote ceremonies since the early 1900s. It still took the U.S. Congress nearly a hundred years to formally legalize the religious use of peyote—and that was only for Native Americans.*

Native Americans had to fight long and hard for their right to use peyote in religious ceremonies. Off and on throughout this century, many peyotists have had to go to court in order to defend their religious rights—and many have spent time in jail for using a sacred plant to pray to their Creator for help and healing. Native Americans definitely earned their right to use peyote as a religious sacrament. The rest of us may have to do the same.

I think that it is imperative that people continue to study and document the potential shamanic, religious, and psychotherapeutic uses of psychedelics. My hope is that, in time, the government will recognize the right of all people to use sacred plants in respectful and responsible ways. In the meantime, those of us who value the religious entheogens must continue to educate people about their appropriate use and to work together for their eventual decriminalization. Some of us may have to stand up and defend our beliefs—just as some early Christians and Native American peyotists had to do—but hopefully the truth will prevail.

We have seen how the perseverance of Native American peyotists eventu-

ally persuaded Congress to pass the AIRFA. And we have seen the example of how, in Brazil, the three hoasca churches worked together—despite philosophical and ritual differences—to protect the religious use of ayahuasca there. So, there is hope.

METZNER: I sometimes ponder what might happen if the three ayahuasca religions of Brazil were to become the three big world religions of the twenty-first century. Some people laugh when I suggest that, but Daime has already become a popular folk religion in Germany and Holland. It is a genuine "religious revitalization" movement. I've heard individuals practicing Daime songs while they are driving in their cars.

Moreover, quite apart from the growth of Daime, the shamanic use of ayahuasca is increasing dramatically. There are many people taking tours to Brazil and Peru, and there are ayahuasca shamans coming up to the U.S. That is bound to have an accumulative cultural effect.

Two thousand years ago, Judaism, Islam, and Christianity all evolved from the same roots within the same ecosystem—the desert. In his book *Nature and Madness,* Paul Sheppard has written about how the desert environment may have shaped the obsessive monotheistic traditions that evolved there. If Daime, UDV, and Barquinia were to become major world religions, we would have a very different worldview. They have evolved out of a very different environment, involving river and rainforest energy, which is all about flowing and growing.

Brazilian culture is very open and accepting of diversity. I think that the spread of ayahuasca ceremonies could also contribute to a much-needed diffusion of Brazilian consciousness into our Western Anglo-Protestant culture. Brazilians don't seem to have any ideological qualms about investigating concepts such as reincarnation, spirit possession, or paranormal phenomena. They take it all in stride. Our culture could certainly benefit from an infusion of flexibility, diversity, and tolerance.

Appendix A

The Psychology
of Ayahuasca

Charles S. Grob, M.D.

THE FIELD OF *ayahuasca* studies poses a challenge to mainstream psychiatry and psychology. Long neglected by Euro-American science, this Amazonian plant hallucinogen concoction known in native Quechua as the "vine of the dead" or "vine of the soul," has recently begun to attract increasing degrees of interest. Over the last several years investigations into the basic psychopharmacology and physiology of this powerful herbal medicine have been initiated. Questions are beginning to be posed examining the potential of ayahuasca to facilitate states of healing. Cross-cultural anthropological perspectives on the import of indigenous belief systems to ayahuasca's mechanism of action are being validated as essential to fully understanding its unique range of effects. Rational science will now need to confront the dilemma of how to comprehend and make sense of an experience that moves beyond the realm of rational, linear thought.

The fields of psychiatry and psychology have never had an appreciable comfort level with the mind states of aboriginal peoples. Native cultures have often been disparaged and the technologies designed to induce ritual trance states either pathologized or ignored. Years past, during a time of psychoanalytic preeminence, the medicine men, or healers, of these aboriginal peoples were judged to be mentally ill (Devereux 1958), their behaviors variably attributed to diagnoses ranging from schizophrenia to hysteria and epilepsy. The primitive medicine man, or shaman, was often identified as a deranged aboriginal tyrant and the wellspring of that psychopathology inflicting the entire tribal group, preventing their elevation into civilized society. Until quite recently the prevailing perception of the aboriginal has been one of the ignorant, deluded and dangerous savage, whose only salvation lay in abandoning the traditions of his ancestors for the customs and beliefs of modern culture. The proposition of taking seriously the plant technologies underlying the collective belief systems found in native shamanism was given little credence by mainstream science and medicine.

Quietly, the tides of change have begun to turn. Heightened interest in the ancient tools of transcendence have surfaced. After decades of silence following the decline and virtual disappearance of hallucinogen research in the 1960s (Grob 1994), a period of revived interest within the fields of anthropology, psychiatry and psychology has arisen. Additional activity, replaying some of the drama of that previous era of investigation, has occurred outside the bounds of formal and credential-bound science. Ethnobotanical explorations in diverse geographic regions have yielded a surprising plethora of psychoactive plants, some with no prior history of cultural identification. Knowledge of potent psychochemical recipes have begun to disseminate, often with the aid of the Internet. Use of plant hallucinogens, in both underground and formal settings, is growing. It is time for post-modern medical science to reawaken and be attentive to this rapidly emerging phenomenon. Beyond the need to assess safety parameters, the full implications to paradigms of healing and reality need to be grappled with.

We are on the threshold of a new era of scientific exploration. The ancient tools of consciousness alteration may yet hold valuable information needed to safely guide our culture into the next century and an uncertain future. For the mainstream fields of psychiatry and psychology, it is time to reopen the question of the value of shamanic ritual experience, and to ex-

plore the ceremonial structures and technologies within which these phenomena are embedded. From the cultural context of our own historical
evolution, we must ask the question, What can we learn from the past and
peoples with vastly different worldviews than our own? One valuable area
of study which may provide answers are the actual psychoactive plant
sacraments used in aboriginal rituals, their botanical identification, chemical constituents, pharmacologic effect, and cross-cultural function. Plant
hallucinogens have a worldwide distribution and pan-historic record of application (Schultes and Hofmann 1992). There are approximately 150 different species of plant hallucinogens, 130 of these being primarily located
in the New World, and only about 20 in Europe. Their role in early cultures is poorly understood, though some have speculated that they played
a pivotal role at the inception of many of the world's major religions (Huxley 1977; Wasson et al. 1986). The areas of the world most richly endowed
with these powerful botanicals are the tropical rain forests, particularly the
Amazon Basin of northwest South America. And the prototype Amazonian
plant hallucinogen concoction is ayahuasca.

What Is Ayahuasca?

There is an important hallucinogenic drink consumed by the native
peoples of the western half of the Amazon valley and by isolated tribes on
the Pacific slopes of the Ecuadoran and Columbian Andes. The primary
plant material used for this botanical brew is the bark of the giant forest
liana *Banisteriopsis caapi*. This ayahuasca, as it is most commonly called, is
prepared by boiling *Banisteriopsis* bark with the leaves of one or more admixture plants, most commonly *Psychotria viridis*. Although some aboriginal tribes have traditions of using *Banisteriopsis* solely, without any
admixture plants, the predominant pattern of use has called for the addition of plants with diverse profiles of chemical constituents and psychoactive effects.

Ayahuasca possesses a unique phytochemistry. When taken alone,
without the *Banisteriopsis,* many of the admixture plants are not psychoactive. Although *Psychotria viridis* is rich in alkaloids of the potent hallucino-

gen dimethyltryptamine (DMT), it is rendered biochemically inactive after oral consumption through inactivation by monoamine oxidase, an enzyme which degrades DMT, along with endogenous neurotransmitters. However, when *Psychotria* is prepared along with *Banisteriopsis,* which has monoamine oxidase inhibiting action, the DMT is actively absorbed, passes the blood-brain barrier, and exerts powerful hallucinogenic effects on the central nervous system. How the native peoples of the Amazon discovered this sophisticated synergistic plant biochemistry is unknown, although the reductionistic explanation asserts that through generations, even centuries, of trial and error sampling of the abundant and diverse tropical flora, the aboriginal inhabitants of the region happened upon this unusual combination. Asking the native peoples themselves, however, yields a very different response. Virtually all of the ayahuasca-using tribes of the Amazon Basin, as well as the modern syncretic churches, who use this plant hallucinogen concoction as a legal psychoactive ritual sacrament, attribute the discovery of ayahuasca, along with the mythological origins of their own idiosyncratic religious belief systems, to a form of divine intervention. However human beings happened to come upon or were directed to this unique phytochemical combination, its discovery was integral to both the development of early native cultures as well as the rise of interest in these sacred plants in our own day.

Biochemically, ayahuasca is a combination of dimethyltryptamine, from the leaves of *Psychotria,* and three harmala alkaloids from *Banisteriopsis* bark, harmine, harmaline and tetrahydroharmine. Dimethyltryptamine has a remarkable structural similarity to the endogenous neurotransmitter serotonin, or 5-hydroxytryptamine. The serotonin system is thought to be the primary neurotransmitter system involved in the activation and modulation of DMT's profound effect upon central nervous system function. The central structural feature of DMT biochemistry is the presence of the indole ring, a characteristic which it shares with serotonin as well as other potent hallucinogens, including lysergic acid diethylamide (LSD). Hallucinogenic tryptamines are present in a variety of plants, including orally active psilocybin mushrooms (the *teonanácatl* of the ancient Aztecs) and the virola snuffs of Amazonian aboriginals. Dimethyltryptamine, as well as its analogue 5-methoxy-dimethyltryptamine, rapidly induce an intense altered state of consciousness of relatively short duration when smoked or snorted intranasally, but are entirely without effect when ingested orally. The harmala alkaloids derived from *Banisteriopsis* are ß-carbolines, which possess potent monoamine oxidase inhibiting (MAOI) action. This MAOI activity allows for a unique profile of biochemical effects, most prominently the activation and augmentation of additive plants. When taken alone, the harmala alkaloids may induce varying degrees of hallucinogenic inebriation, and are utilized ritually for this purpose by particular native tribes. The characteristically bitter taste of ayahuasca, along with its nauseating and emetic effects, are attributable to these harmala alkaloids.

Historical Antecedents

Archeological evidence supports the existence of the ritual use of plant hallucinogens by native peoples of the New World, long predating the arrival of the European explorers and colonists (Adovasio and Fry 1976; Torres et al. 1991). By the sixteenth century, however, particularly in the more tropical regions of Central and South America, with their greater abundance of psychoactive botanicals, the aboriginal utilization of native pharmacopeia began to evoke a harsh and punitive reaction. The occupying Spaniards and Portuguese, possessors now of most of the New World's rain forests, brutally persecuted and exploited native cultures (Taussig 1987). Observing the utilization of sacred plants to induce an ecstatic intoxication, and identifying the central role they played in aboriginal religion and ritual, these new European overlords harshly condemned their use. Hernando Ruiz de Alarcon, an early Spanish chronicler of native customs, described how the plants "when drunk deprive of the senses, because it is very powerful, and by this means they communicate with the devil, because he talks to them when they are deprived of judgement with the said drink, and deceive them with different hallucinations, and they attribute it to a god they say is inside the seed" (Guerra 1971). Condemned by the Holy Inquisition in 1616, the ceremonial use of plant hallucinogens by aboriginal peoples of the New World survived only by going deeply underground, remaining hidden from the hostile and rapacious European-imposed dominant culture.

Knowledge of ayahuasca use by native peoples of the Amazon was first recorded in the seventeenth century when Jesuit priests described the existence of "diabolical potions," prepared from forest vines by the native people of Peru (Ott 1994). There was no additional mention in the collective literature until the mid-nineteenth century when Richard Spruce, an English botanist doing fieldwork in the Amazon, identified the bark of a liana as the central substance in the legendary aboriginal *caapi*, or *yagé*. Later, when subjected to modern biochemical analysis, this specimen of Spruce's, having been kept for over one hundred years in storage at a British museum, was identified as a sample of *Banisteriopsis* containing harmala alkaloids. The first written report describing ayahuasca from a contemporaneous source was in 1858 by Manuel Villavicencio, an Ecuadoran geographer, who studied tribal groups in the Rio Napo area of Ecuador. Intrigued by the use of yagé in rituals, Villavicencio sought the opportunity to investigate first-hand the subjective effects of this beverage. He would later describe "in a few moments it begins to produce the most rare phenomena. Its action appears to excite the nervous system; all the senses liven up and all faculties awaken; they feel vertigo and spinning in the head, followed by a sensation of being lifted into the air and beginning an aerial journey; the possessed begins in the first moments to see the most delicious apparitions, in conformity with his ideas and knowledge; the savages [apparently the Záparo of eastern Ecuador] say that they see gorgeous lakes, forests covered with fruit, the prettiest birds who communicate to them the nicest and the most favorable things they want to hear, and other beautiful things relating to their savage life. When this instant passes they begin to see terrible horrors out to devour them, their first flight ceases and they descend to earth to combat the terrors who communicate to them all adversities and misfortunes awaiting them. . . . As for myself I can say for a fact that when I've taken ayahuasca I've experienced dizziness, then an aerial journey in which I recall perceiving the most gorgeous views, great cities, lofty towers, beautiful parks, and other extremely attractive objects; then I imagined myself to be alone in a forest and assaulted by a number of terrible beings from which I defended myself; thereafter I had the strong sensation of sleep. . . ." (Villavicencio 1858; Harner 1973a).

Anthropological Perspective

Among the diverse native peoples of the Amazon basin, ayahuasca has been known by a variety of names, including *caapi, yagé, natéma, mihi, kahi, pinde* and *dapa.* Ayahuasca is perceived as a magic intoxicant, of divine origin, which facilitates release of the soul from its corporeal confinement, allowing it to wander free and return to the body at will, carrying with it information of vital import (Schultes and Hofmann 1992). Among native peoples, ayahuasca was traditionally used for purposes of magic and religious ritual, divination, sorcery, and the treatment of disease (Dobkin de Rios 1972). Living among the Cashinahua of the Peruvian Amazon, the anthropologist Kenneth Kensinger (1973) identified ayahuasca-induced visions as integral to the genesis of volitional behavior. These visions are perceived as the experiences of an individual's "dream spirit," which has access to knowledge contained in the supernatural realms. Kensinger has described how the Cashinahua use ayahuasca as a means of receiving information not available through the normal channels of communication, which, along with additional information accessed through other means, constitutes the basis for personal action. For the Cashinahua, however, taking ayahuasca is an unpleasant and even fearful experience, which is resorted to only when such revelations from the spirit world are urgently needed.

For the Jivaro Indians of the Ecuadoran Amazon, the supernatural realm, which can only be accessed through the door of the ayahuasca-induced experience, is seen as the true reality, whereas normal waking life is simply an illusion. Michael Harner, an anthropologist who has lived among and studied the Jivaro, has understood the importance of the ayahuasca experience itself in order to fully grasp the aboriginal mindset. Although traditional anthropological observers have typically assumed a passive role in compiling and recording native habits and customs, Harner elected to undergo a first-hand encounter with the object of his study.

Harner has described how "for several hours after drinking the brew, I found myself, although awake, in a world literally beyond my wildest dreams. I met bird-headed people, as well as dragon-like creatures who explained that they were the true gods of this world. I enlisted the services of other spirit helpers in attempting to fly through the far reaches of the Galaxy. Transported into a trance where the supernatural seemed natural, I realized that anthropologists, including myself, had profoundly underestimated the importance of the drug in affecting native ideology" (Harner 1973b).

Integral to the content of the realm of ayahuasca-induced visions is the cultural context in which they occur. Throughout the tropical rain forests of South America, the traditional ayahuasca-using tribal people have many shared common cultural elements as well as similar contextual themes for their mythologies and ayahuasca-induced experiences. Indeed, some anthropological observers have asserted that it is virtually impossible to separate the nature of the ayahuasca experience from its cultural context (Harner 1973a). Through contacting the supernatural realm of their ancestors, as well as their mythological deities and spirits, the ritual use of ayahuasca has served to bind the communities of disparate individuals into a cohesive collective culture. Culturally syntonic visions are induced by shamanic manipulation of set and setting to provide revelation, blessings, healing and ontological security for those using such sacramental plants (Grob and Dobkin de Rios 1992). Within traditional contexts, shamanic initiation into the world of plant hallucinogens, including ayahuasca, have included long preparations associated with strict self-discipline, including prolonged social isolation, sexual abstinence, and diets free of meat, salt, sugar and alcohol. The collective ingestion of these ceremonial sacraments by the adult members of the community achieves an amplified degree of social cohesion and identity which has been characterized by Mircea Eliade as a periodic symbolic regression to the "powerful time" of mythical origin (Eliade 1964). Ultimately, the intent of the collective ayahuasca sessions is not necessarily to evoke visions from each tribal individual's unconscious, but rather to assimilate and absorb the unconscious biographical personality structure into the cultural patterns of the visionary motifs (Andritzky 1989).

Contemporary Contexts

Since the time of European conquest and colonization of the New World several hundred years ago, the original native peoples of the Amazon basin have been all but eradicated. First through policies of virtual genocide, enslavement, and forced labor (Taussig 1987), then through the rampant dissemination of infectious disease, and later through the process of gradual acculturation to European values, culture, and religion, aboriginal customs and belief systems have barely survived to the present day. Only in the most remote regions of the rain forest have isolated tribes been able to avoid the relentless onslaught of modern culture, whether it has been from capitalist or missionary motive. Consequently, the traditional use of ayahuasca by native peoples has virtually disappeared, replaced by belief systems and forms of worship antithetical to the ways of their ancestors. By bringing such trappings of modern civilization to the world of the heathen, often in the form of missionary medical aid, the aboriginal people of the Amazon have been encouraged, sometimes gently and sometimes through coercion, to abandon their traditional use of ayahuasca. Nevertheless, knowledge of this extraordinary herbal concoction, representative of what Schultes and Hofmann (1992) have termed these "plants of the Gods," has survived. In diverse forms, reflecting their modern cultural contexts, the use of ayahuasca for purposes of healing and religious worship has persisted to our present day.

As the use of ayahuasca was central to conceptualizing and treating illness among native peoples, so this model for healing has persisted among mestizo, or mixed race, populations throughout the Amazon basin. The anthropologist Marlene Dobkin de Rios has studied the phenomena of urban mestizo healing in the Peruvian tropical rain forest city of Iquitos (Dobkin de Rios 1972). Her work has described not only a particular context in which the use of ayahuasca has persisted, but also how it has served a protective function against the stressors of modern life. Demoralized by the shock of acculturative forces, mestizo inhabitants of Iquitos suffer from high rates of stress-induced anxiety and associated psychosomatic disorders. The use of ayahuasca, as supervised by mestizo healers, is incorporated into complex ritual healing ceremonies. Such a model for ayahuasca healing is most efficacious with illnesses which are believed to be magical in origin. The primary function of taking ayahuasca in this context is to diagnose the magical cause of illness, as well as to deflect and neutralize the evil spirits or magic which are believed to be responsible for particular types of illness. Within the context of a collective belief system which still maintains a conviction that such supernatural realms do exist, this model for ayahuasca healing among modern-day Amazonian mestizos appears to function with a fair degree of success (Dobkin de Rios 1984).

Another model for ayahuasca healing has been developed in the Peruvian upper Amazon province of San Martin. The Takiwasi Center, created in the mid-1980s by a group of French and Peruvian physicians and healers, was inspired both by knowledge of the salutary effects of the legendary vine and the pressing need to identify an effective treatment for the rapidly increasing problem of coca paste addiction. A cheap intermediary between the raw coca plant and refined cocaine, coca paste is a highly addictive drug which has spread throughout the coca-cultivating and cocaine-producing regions of South America. Conventional treatment models for coca paste addiction have largely proved ineffectual, thus compounding this public health dilemma. Studying models for shamanic healing among extant native peoples, the Takiwasi group has developed their own involved structure for the ayahuasca-facilitated treatment of drug addiction (Mabit 1988; Mabit et al. 1995). The phenomena of Takiwasi may serve as an early example of the identification and use of ayahuasca for purposes of healing refractory conditions by physicians trained in modern medicine.

During the twentieth century the use of ayahuasca has been incorporated into the ritual practices of organized syncretic churches in Brazil. The first such ayahuasca church, the Santo Daime, began in the 1930s in the Brazilian Amazon region of Acre (Groisman and Sell 1995). Founded originally among mixed race *caboclos* and rubber tappers, the Santo Daime subsequently spread among middle-class populations throughout Brazil and ultimately abroad. The primary centers of Santo Daime activity included the founding of several self-sustaining communities in isolated regions of the Amazonian rain forest.

In the early 1960s, also in Acre state, an independent ayahuasca-using religion was founded by Jose Gabriel da Costa, who had acquired knowledge of this powerful sacramental plant preparation while working as a rubber tapper in the rain forests of Bolivia. Returning to his native Brazil, Mestre Gabriel, as he came to be called by his disciples, founded the Centre Espirita Beneficente União do Vegetal (UDV). Spreading primarily to urban areas, the UDV became the largest and most organized of the ayahuasca churches, ultimately establishing its headquarters in the Brazilian capital city of Brasilia (Ott 1993). The UDV was also primarily responsible for the successful petition to the Brazilian government to remove ayahuasca from the list of banned substances. Establishing an extraordinary precedent, the Brazilian government in 1987 declared ayahuasca to be a legal substance when used within the context of religious practice, thus becoming the first nation worldwide in almost 1600 years to allow the use of plant hallucinogens for spiritual purposes by its nonindigenous inhabitants.

Over the past decade knowledge and use of ayahuasca has spread throughout Europe and North America. This activity has come primarily from two directions. The Brazilian ayahuasca churches, the Santo Daime in particular, have established centers in many cities across Europe, with greatest activity in Spain, Holland and Germany. The UDV has been much more circumspect and cautious, however, maintaining a relatively low profile and avoiding unnecessary and unwelcome media attention. This pattern has continued in the United States, particularly on the West Coast, where in recent years the Santo Daime has held a number of "works," generally open events with minimal screening or preparation of participants, whereas UDV activities, under direction from the centralized church hierarchy in Brazil, have limited participation only to formal UDV members and individuals who had been previously introduced to the plant sacrament and ritual.

Increasing interest in the ayahuasca studies of North American scholars and scientists has also begun to spur new activities in this area. In particular, the work of the autodidact writer and underground investigator Jonathan Ott has yielded a rich harvest of information. In books (Ott 1993;

Ott 1994a; and articles (Ott 1994b; Ott 1999), Ott has, in voluminous detail, described the varieties of plant and synthetic substances with chemical properties similar to those of the primary plants of Amazonian ayahuasca, *Banisteriopsis* and *Psychotria*. These ayahuasca analogues, plants containing ß-carboline harmala alkaloids, including *Peganum harmala* (Syrian rue), along with additional plants rich in tryptamines (e.g., *Anadenanthera colubrina*, *Mimosa hostilis* and *Philaris arundinacea*), provide rich, alternative non-tropical sources of powerful plant hallucinogenic experience. With the virtually worldwide and previously largely unknown distribution of such ayahuasca analogues, Ott has provided the blueprint to what he has termed the pan-Gaean entheogenic revival (Ott 1994a). Similarly, laboratory analogues for ayahuasca, combinations of synthetic dimethyltryptamine, harmine, and harmaline, have been described which approximate the subjective effects of the prototype plant beverage. This pharmahuasca, as identified by Ott and others (Ott 1999; Callaway 1994), possesses the extraordinary capacity, along with the diverse plant analogues, to replicate the legendary ayahuasca experience for large numbers of "psychonauts" without proximity or access to the tropical plants. The implications of this phenomena, in an age of increasingly rapid dissemination of information, make the medical and scientific examination of ayahuasca all the more compelling.

What Is the Ayahuasca Experience?

As is the case with all hallucinogens, the ayahuasca experience is profoundly affected by the extrapharmacological factors of set and setting (Bravo and Grob 1989). Intention, preparation, and structure of the session are all integral to the content and outcome of any encounter with hallucinogens, a clear distinction from virtually all other psychotropic agents. The diligent attention to these factors are known to be integral to the shamanic model of altered states of consciousness, minimizing risks and enhancing the likelihood of salutary results. The failure to adequately comprehend and adhere to the wisdom behind these time-tested safeguards, on the other hand, often leads to the unfortunate consequences frequently observed within the context of contemporary recreational drug use and abuse (Grob and Dobkin de Rios 1992; Dobkin de Rios and Grob 1994).

Altered states of consciousness, including those induced by hallucinogens, possess a variety of common elements (Ludwig 1969; Dobkin de Rios 1972). Before examining those features more closely identified with the ayahuasca experience, these shared properties merit review. The ten general characteristics understood to be virtually universal to such altered state experience include:

1. Alterations in Thinking. To varying degrees, subjective changes in concentration, attention, memory and judgment may be induced in the acute state, along with a possible diminution or expansion of reflective awareness.
2. Altered Time Sense. The sense of time and chronology may become altered, inducing a subjective feeling of timelessness, or the experience of time either accelerating or decelerating. Time may be experienced as infinite, or infinitesimal in duration.
3. Fear of Loss of Control. An individual may experience a fear of losing his hold on reality or his sense of self-control. In reaction, increased resistance to the experience may occur, causing an amplification of underlying anxiety. If there is a positive cultural conditioning and understanding of the experience, mystical and positive transcendent states may ensue.
4. Changes in Emotional Expression. Along with reduction in volitional or conscious control, intense emotional reactivity may occur, ranging from ecstasy to despair.
5. Changes in Body Image. Alterations in body image are frequently reported, often associated with dissolution of boundaries between self and others and states of depersonalization and derealization where the usual sense of one's own reality is temporarily lost or changed. Such experiences may be regarded

as strange and frightening, or as mystical, oceanic states of cosmic unity, particularly when sustained within the context of belief systems conditioned for spiritual emergent encounters.

6. Perceptual Alterations. Increased visual imagery, hyperacuteness of perceptions and overt hallucinations may occur. The content of these perceptual alterations are influenced by cultural expectations, group influences and individual wish-fulfillment fantasies. They may reflect the psychodynamic expression of underlying fears or conflicts, or simple neurophysiologic mechanisms inducing geometric patterns and alterations of light, colors and shapes. Synesthesia, the transformation of one form of sensory experience into another, such as seeing auditory stimuli, may be experienced.

7. Changes in Meaning or Significance. While in a powerful altered state of consciousness, some individuals manifest a propensity to attach special meaning or significance to their subjective experiences, ideas or perceptions. An experience of great insight or profound sense of meaning may occur, their significance ranging from genuine wisdom to self-imposed delusion.

8. Sense of the Ineffable. Because of the uniqueness of the subjective experience associated with these states and their divergence from ordinary states of consciousness, individuals often have great difficulty communicating the essence of their experience to those who have never had such an encounter.

9. Feelings of Rejuvenation. Many individuals emerging from a profoundly altered state of consciousness report a new sense of hope, rejuvenation and rebirth. Such transformed states may be short-term, or conversely, may lead to sustained positive adjustments in mood and outlook.

10. Hyper-suggestibility. While in the throes of altered state experience, individuals experience an enhanced susceptibility to accept or respond uncritically to specific statements. Nonspecific cues, reflecting cultural belief systems or group expectation,

may similarly assume directives of weighty importance. The position of shaman, or session facilitator, particularly within the
context of hallucinogen use, consequently becomes a role with
great vested responsibility, as individual participants are highly
susceptible to verbal and nonverbal input directed towards
them. The content and outcome of such altered states experiences are often directly attributable to the integrity and skill of
the leader.

Reports of specific ayahuasca effects vary greatly depending upon the
cultural context, which may range from traditional native Amazonian ritual, to mestizo healing ceremony, to syncretic religious structure, to in-
quisitive Euro-American psychonautic exploration. The Tukano tribe of
the Columbian Amazonia separate the ayahuasca experience into three
stages. The first stage, which may begin within minutes of ingestion, induces the characteristic gastrointestinal reaction of nausea, emesis, and
diarrhea, along with sweating, a sense of "flying," and the visual perception
of vivid, kaleidoscopic array of brightly colored lights and geometric patterns. During the second phase of ayahuasca intoxication for the Tukano,
the perception of brightly colored geometric patterns start to fade, while
the sensation of flight into deep internal space intensifies along with an
envisioning of three-dimensional forms of mythological and "monstrous"
animals. The third and final stage involves the deepening of hallucinations,
along with a progression into calmer and more peaceful visions and thought
associations (Reichel-Dolmatoff 1975; Schultes and Winkelman 1995).
Commonalities of the ayahuasca visionary experience among diverse
aboriginal groups of the tropical rain forests of South America have been
described (Harner 1973b). Shared elements include:

1. The perception of the separation of the soul from the physical
   body associated with the sensation of flying. This astral voyage
   persists for the duration of the effects of the ayahuasca, after
   which the soul re-enters the body. With some tribal people, the

soul leaves the body in the form of a bird, which flies to some pre-determined destination. A sensation of vertigo, or spinning, is often experienced.

2. Visions of snakes and jaguars, along with other predatory animals of the rain forest. Snakes and giant anacondas in particular populate the visions of native people. On some occasions, the ayahuasca voyager perceives himself to be attacked and consumed by these reptilian marauders, whereas at other times it is the snakes which are ingested. Confrontations with such rain forest predators may be empowering to the traveler, allowing him to forge an alliance with them as powerful shamanic spirit animals which may assist him in his journeys and battles in the supernatural realm.

3. The sense of contact with supernatural realms. Visions are experienced of deities and/or demons, consistent with the shamanic belief systems of native voyagers. For native Indians influenced by the entreaties of missionary Christianity, yet who have maintained their traditions of ritual ayahuasca use, visitations to heaven and the realms of hell are reported.

4. Visions of distant persons, cities, and landscapes, which are understood by native Indians as clairvoyant experience. Such sensations of "seeing" events and locations far removed in place and time are utilized for purposes ranging from identifying wherein the forest plentiful game may be available for the hunt, to inquiring about the health and well-being of relatives or friends, to practicing the many forms of sorcery which exist among aboriginal Amazonian tribes.

5. The sensation of "seeing" the detailed re-enactment of recent unsolved crimes, or of identifying through visions the shaman responsible for bewitching a sick or dying person. Among many tribal groups, illness is understood to be caused by the actions of bewitchment, whereas the healing process relies upon the identification of the shaman responsible for the condition. Ayahuasca divination may address such tasks as identifying the perpetrators of recent homicides or thefts, discovering the plans of enemy at-

tacks, predicting the imminent arrival of strangers, the adjudication of quarrels or disputes and the investigation of whether spouses are faithful.

Modern observers have reported a range of experience reflective of their own cultural context, although rain forest motifs common to aboriginal peoples are often in evidence. Reports of predatory animals, particularly snakes, are described not only within the tropical setting of mestizo healing (Dobkin de Rios 1971; Flores and Lewis 1978), but by sophisticated inhabitants of urban areas far removed from the forest as well (Naranjo 1973). Depending upon the belief system of participants, both collective and individual, ayahuasca visionary experiences are shaped. Within the context of the Brazilian syncretic churches, for example, it is not uncommon for practitioners to encounter visions incorporating elements of their religious mythology, and to interpret these events according to church precept (Groisman and Sell 1995; Grob et al. 1996).

Although an element of unpredictability is inherent even with experienced users (Mabit et al. 1995), the likelihood of being overwhelmed by frightening visions is enhanced when individuals venture into the realm of ayahuasca with neither adequate preparation nor a ritual structure designed to contain and channel the experience. In 1960, anticipating the psychonautic exploration of many of his countrymen several decades later, the American poet Allen Ginsberg ventured into the Peruvian Amazon town of Pucallpa in search of the legendary yagé experience. Accessing a concoction of ayahuasca from a local *curandero,* or mestizo healer, Ginsberg ingested the brew. Describing his experience the next day in a letter written to his friend William Burroughs, Ginsberg wrote:

First I began to realize my worry about the mosquitoes or vomiting was silly as there was the great stake of life and Death—I felt faced by Death, my skull in my beard on pallet and porch rolling back and forth and settling finally as if in reproduction of the last physical move I make before settling into real death—got nauseous, rushed out and began vomiting, all covered with snakes, like a Snake Seraph, colored serpents in aureole all around my body, I felt like a snake vomiting out the universe. . . . I was frightened and simply lay there with wave after wave of death—fear, fright, rolling over me till I could hardly stand it, didn't want to take refuge in rejecting it as illusion, for it was too real and too familiar—especially as if rehearsal of Last Minute Death my head rolling back and forth on the blanket and finally settling in last position of stillness and hopeless resignation to God knows what Fate—for my being—felt completely lost strayed soul—outside of contact with some Thing that seemed present—finally had a sense that I might face the Question there and then, and choose to die and understand—and leave my body to be found in the morning (Burroughs and Ginsberg 1963).

As is the case with other hallucinogens, ayahuasca has the innate potential to plunge those who might sample its range of experience into the depths of hell or, conversely, into the exalted planes of the celestial realms. Contrasting with the terrifying existential nightmarish quality of Ginsberg's experience is the report of Heinz Kusel, a trader living among the Chama Indians of northeast Peru during the late 1940s. After two unpleasant episodes following ingestion of ayahuasca, Kusel decided to undergo another attempt at achieving that level of experience he had heard about from local inhabitants. Describing the last of these three experiences taken under the supervision of Nolorbe, his native guide, Kusel would subsequently write that:

the images were not casual, accidental or imperfect, but fully organized to the last detail of highly complex, consistent, yet forever changing designs. . . . I was very conscious at the time of an inexplicable sensation of intimacy with the visions. They were mine and concerned only me. I remember an Indian telling me that whenever he drank ayahuasca, he had such beautiful visions that he used to put his hands over his eyes for fear somebody might steal them. I felt the same way. . . . The color scheme became a harmony of dark browns and greens. Naked dancers appeared turning slowly in spiral

movements. Spots of brassy lights played on their bodies which gave them the texture of polished stones. Their faces were inclined and hidden in deep shadows. Their coming into existence in the center of the vision coincided with the rhythm of Nolorbe's song, and they advanced forward and to the sides, turning slowly. I longed to see their faces. At last the whole field of vision was taken up by a single dancer with inclined face covered by a raised arm. As my desire to see the face became unendurable, it appeared suddenly in full close-up with closed eyes. I know that when the extraordinary face opened them, I experienced a satisfaction of a kind I had never known. It was the visual solution of a personal riddle (Kusel 1965).

Neuropsychiatric Research with Ayahuasca

Scientific and medical interest in ayahuasca long predated recent activities in the field. During the 1920s and 1930s, European and American pharmacologists and physicians began to pay attention to the exotic plant drug concoction from the tropical rain forests of South America. Working with specimens of *Banisteriopsis* bark, believed at that time to be the sole constituent of the legendary jungle drink, the renowned German research psychopharmacologist, Louis Lewin, in his final project before his death, succeeded in isolating one of the active alkaloids of ayahuasca, harmine, which he initially named banisterine (Lewin 1929). At Lewin's suggestion, the neurologist Kurt Beringer explored the effects of banisterine, also known as telepathine, in reference to the legendary properties of the jungle vine, in the treatment of Parkinson's Disease. Administering the drug to fifteen patients with postencephalitic Parkinsonism, Beringer reported the dramatic improvement of the classic symptoms of rigidity and akinesia (Beringer 1928). Although the use of banisterine in the treatment of Parkinson's Disease would ultimately be replaced by other drugs, most notably L-dopa, this application provides an early reference point for the discovery of medicinal uses of ayahuasca by modern investigators (Sanchez-Ramos 1991).

Although notable gains have been made in the past two decades exploring the basic biochemistry of ayahuasca (McKenna et al. 1998), formal psychiatric research investigations have not been pursued until recently. In part attributed to the thirty-year-old taboo against pursuing sanctioned psychiatric research with hallucinogens (Grob 1994), and in part because of the long-standing resistance to investigating primary plant products by modern science, the seemingly remote rain forest plant concoction ayahuasca has until now received virtually no attention by established medical scientists. The enthusiasm among European physicians earlier in this century following the breakthrough discoveries of Lewin and Beringer now long forgotten, medical-psychiatric ayahuasca investigation had long slumbered.

Even during the period of the 1950s and 1960s, when interest in the basic properties and even therapeutic potential of hallucinogens was considered a valid pursuit, little interest in conducting investigations of ayahuasca was in evidence. There was some activity, however, directed at exploring the effects of synthetic harmala alkaloids. Working with synthetic harmine, early investigators expressed doubt as to its inherent psychoactivity (Turner et al. 1955; Pennes and Hoch 1957). The first to establish that harmala alkaloids possessed hallucinogenic activity was the Chilean psychiatrist and psychopharmacologist, Claudio Naranjo. Examining the basic psychogenic properties of harmaline, Naranjo identified the hallucinogenic threshold to be at dosage levels above 1 milligram per kilogram (mg/kg) intravenously, or 4 mg/kg orally. Contrasting its effects to the classic hallucinogens LSD and mescaline, Naranjo described that "the typical reaction to harmaline is a closed-eye contemplation of vivid imagery . . . which is in contrast to the ecstatic heavens or dreadful hells of other hallucinogens" (Naranjo, 1967). Naranjo found the effects of harmaline to be relatively calming and subtle, his subjects reporting relaxed states of philosophical and religious contemplation, without emotional turmoil. In 8 of 30 patients to whom he administered the drug, pronounced ameliorations of neurotic symptoms were reported (Naranjo 1973). Although significant in establishing harmaline's basic psychoactivity, Naranjo was not able to account for the powerful affective and perceptual altering experiences described in reports of the effects of ayahuasca. Subsequent investigators would resolve this question by identifying that harmaline is not only present in relative trace amounts in ayahuasca—far exceeded quantitatively by harmine—but that ayahuasca is likely to possess its potent hallucinatory properties on the basis of admixture plants included in its preparation (McKenna et al. 1984; Ott 1993).

There exist in nature over seventy-five plants which have been used by indigenous peoples in the preparation of ayahuasca (Bianchi and Samorini, 1993). Most commonly, admixture plants containing tryptamine derivatives, in particular N,N-dimethyltryptamine (DMT), are combined with ß-carboline harmala alkaloids (McKenna and Towers 1984) to induce the powerful hallucinogenic effect. During the 1950s and 1960s laboratory and clinical studies examined the psychopharmacologic effects of tryptamines, primarily as a probe to determine the neurobiologic basis of mental disease (Turner and Merlis 1959). Efforts to associate the presence of endogenous DMT with mental illness, however, did not prove successful owing to the detection of tryptamine derivatives in the body fluids of both patients and control subjects. Naturally occurring DMT has been detected in tissues and body fluids of several mammalian species, including humans (Callaway 1995). A close association between DMT and the serotonin (5-hydroxytryptamine) neurotransmitter system has also been identified. Indeed, endogenous production of DMT was noted to proceed directly from tryptamine. More recently, a novel hypothesis has been proposed which suggests that the natural occurrence and function of tryptamines within the human central nervous system can be explained by their role promoting the visual phenomenon of dream sleep (Callaway 1988). Similar to the mechanism of ayahuasca action, increased levels of endogenous ß-carbolines during sleep are presumed to facilitate activity of methylated tryptamines by blocking their metabolism.

During the 1990s, a program of clinical investigation of DMT in normal volunteer subjects was pursued at the University of New Mexico. The first hallucinogen research study to receive FDA approval after a greater than two decade hiatus, the team of R.J. Strassman and colleagues at the University of New Mexico studied basic pharmacologic, physiologic and psychologic effects of DMT in normal volunteer subjects (Strassman et al.

1994). When administered graded doses of intravenous DMT in the clinical laboratory setting, subjects reported seeing with their eyes closed rapidly moving, brightly colored visual displays of images. Subjectively, they described experiencing a lessening of control initiated by a brief but overwhelming "rush," which led to a dissociated state where euphoria alternated or coexisted with anxiety. The dosage range for activation of the hallucinogenic state was determined to be between 0.2 mg/kg and 0.4 mg/kg intravenous DMT. At the dosage levels at or above 0.4 mg/kg subjects uniformly reported feeling overwhelmed by the intensity and speed of onset of the experience.

The Hoasca Project

The first, and to date only, formal psychiatric research investigation of ayahuasca took place in the Brazilian Amazon city of Manaus in 1993. A multinational collaborative study, the Hoasca Project, examined biochemical (Callaway et al. 1994), pharmacological (Callaway et al. 1996), physiological (Callaway et al. 1999) and psychiatric (Grob et al. 1996) perspectives. The primary objective of these investigations was to establish a core of qualitative and quantitative data on the psychopharmacology of ayahuasca, which could establish relative safety profiles for human consumption as well as provide the foundation for future studies (McKenna et al. 1998). Given the legally protected status of ayahuasca in Brazil, a unique environment for the sanctioned investigation of hoasca (the Portuguese transliteration of ayahuasca) was available. Conducted with the full cooperation of the syncretic religious church, União do Vegetal (UDV), the Hoasca Project has established a model and precedent for the biomedical investigation of ayahuasca in its natural setting.

Method: For the purposes of this pilot investigation, fifteen long-term users of ayahuasca and fifteen matched controls were recruited. Ayahuasca-using subjects were all members of the UDV, of at least ten years standing, who consumed ayahausca in religious rituals at a frequency of at least two times monthly. Control subjects were matched along all demographic parameters, with the exception that they did not belong to the UDV and had never consumed ayahuasca. A variety of parameters were utilized to assess past and current levels of psychological function. Both ayahuasca-experienced subjects and normal controls were administered structured psychiatric diagnostic interviews (Composite International Diagnostic Interview [CIDI]), lifestory interviews, personality testing (Tridimensional Personality Questionnaire [TPQ]), and neuropsychological testing (WHO–UCLA Auditory Verbal Learning Test). Ayahuasca-experienced subjects were asked to fill out an additional questionnaire (Hallucinogen Rating Scale [HRS]) following an experimental ayahuasca session. Each of the ayahuasca subjects were also interviewed utilizing a semistructured format designed to ascertain their life stories. In addition to this psychiatric investigation, a research methodology designed to evaluate serotonin biochemistry, through the examination of platelet serotonin receptor activity in both experimental and control subjects, was pursued. Additional biological investigations included tryptamine and harmala pharmacokinetics as well as acute physiological and neuroendocrine effects of ayahuasca in long-term users.

Results: Diagnostic and life-story interviews identified appreciable past psychiatric and substance abuse histories in the UDV subjects prior to their entry into the ayahuasca church, including 73% with histories of significant alcohol use, 33% with alcohol binging associated with violent behavior, 27% with stimulant abuse and 53% with tobacco dependence. For all of these subjects, however, past psychopathology had resolved following initiation and regular attendance at ayahuasca ceremonies. Personality testing identified significant differences between the ayahuasca-using and nonusing groups. These included measures of novelty seeking, with UDV members described as being more reflective, rigid, loyal, stoic, slow-tempered, frugal, orderly, and persistent, and also scoring higher on measures of social desirability and emotional maturity than controls. Ayahuasca-using subjects were also distinguished from controls on the harm avoidance domain as being more confident, relaxed, optimistic, carefree, uninhibited, outgoing, and energetic. Overall, the UDV ayahuasca-using group scored higher on traits of hyperthymia, cheerfulness, stubbornness and overconfidence than their nonusing counterparts. Baseline neuropsychological testing also revealed differences between the two groups, with the long-term ayahuasca users demonstrating significantly higher scores on measures of concentration and short-term memory. The final psychological instrument, employed on ayahuasca subjects only, was the Hallucinogen Rating Scale, designed to correlate the intensity and phenomenology of the subjective state with known measures of intravenous dimethyltryptamine (Strassman et al. 1994). In this study of ayahuasca, scores in the 0.1 to 0.2 mg/kg range of intravenous DMT were recorded.

Life-story interviews were employed to gather additional personal histories of UDV subjects prior to ayahuasca initiation, the nature of their first ayahuasca experience, and an account of how their lives had changed following entry into the syncretic ayahuasca church. For most of the interview sample, their lives before entry into the UDV were described as impulsive, disrespectful, angry, aggressive, oppositional, rebellious, irresponsible, alienated, and unsuccessful. Many of them had profound initial encounters with ayahuasca. A common theme for their visionary experience was the perception of being on a self-destructive path which would ultimately lead to an ignominious end unless they radically reformed their personal conduct and orientation. Descriptions of these frightening visions included "I had a vision of myself in a car going to a party. There was a terrible accident and I could see myself die." "I was at a carnival, on a carousel, going around and around without ever stopping. I didn't know how to get off. I was very frightened." "I could see where I was going with the life I was leading. I could see myself ending up in a hospital, in a prison, in a cemetery." "I saw myself arrested and taken to prison. They were going to execute me for a horrible crime I had committed." While in the throes of their nightmarish visionary experience, several of the subjects reported encountering the founder of the UDV, Mestre Gabriel, who would deliver them from their terrors: "I saw these horrible, ugly animals. They attacked me. My body was disassembled, different parts were lying all over the ground. Then I saw the Mestre. He told me what I would need to do to put all my body parts back together." "I ran through the forest terrified that I was going to die. Then I saw the Mestre. He looked at me. I was bathed in his light. I knew I would be okay." "I was in a canoe, out of control, going down the river. I thought I would die. But then I saw Mestre Gabriel in a canoe in front of me. I knew that as long as I stayed with the Mestre I was safe."

All of the long-term ayahuasca-using subjects reported during the life-story interviews that they had undergone a personal transformation following entry into the UDV and regular participation in ritual ayahuasca use. In addition to entirely discontinuing cigarette, alcohol and recreational drug use, they reported a radical restructuring of their personal conduct an value systems. One subject described how: "I used to not care about anybody, but now I know about responsibility. Every day I work on being a good father, a good husband, a good friend, a good worker. I try to do what I can to help others. . . . I have learned to be calmer, more self confident, more accepting of others. . . . I have gone through a transformation." Subjects emphasized the importance of "practicing good deeds," watching one's words, and having respect for nature. Subjects also reported sustained improvement in memory and concentration, persistent positive mood states, fulfillment in day-to-day interactions, and a sense of purpose, meaning and coherence to their lives.

All of the subjects interviewed unequivocally attributed the positive changes in their lives to their experiences within the UDV and their participation in the ritual ingestion of ayahuasca. They described ayahuasca as a catalyst for their moral and psychological evolution. They also insisted, though, that it was not necessarily the ayahuasca alone which was responsible, but rather partaking of the ayahuasca within the ritual context of the UDV ceremonial structure. Criticism of other Brazilian groups which were said to use ayahuasca in less focused and less controlled settings, was expressed by some of the subjects. The UDV was portrayed as a "vessel" that enabled them to safely navigate the often turbulent states of consciousness induced by ayahuasca. They described the UDV as their "mother . . . family . . . house of friends," providing them with "guidance and orientation" and allowing them to walk the "straight path." They emphasized the importance of "união," or union, of the plants and of the people. Without the structure of the UDV, these subjects asserted, ayahuasca experiences may be unpredictable and lead to an inflated sense of self. Within the "house of the UDV," however, the ayahuasca-induced state is controlled and directed "down the path of simplicity and humility."

Discussion: The Hoasca Project has been the first formal psychobiologic investigation of the legendary Amazonian sacrament. Psychological profiles of long-term members of the Brazilian ayahuasca church, União do Vegetal, reveal high levels of function compared to normal controls, including healthier personality measures, superior neuropsychological function. Whether these findings are attributable to the direct effects of ritual ayahuasca ingestion or whether they were self-selecting factors for affiliating with such a process to begin with cannot be determined, given the methodological limitations of this pilot investigation, nevertheless a strong preliminary case can be made for ayahuasca's salutary effects when utilized in such a context. A key factor when examining the apparent outcome of frequent hallucinogen, or ayahausca, use is the set and setting, and the role of suggestibility. For the subjects studied, the syncretic church they belonged to provided a protective and supportive community, as is often the case with all forms of religion. What might mark the phenomenon of the ayahuasca church as distinct, however, is the utilization of a powerful plant hallucinogen as a psychoactive religious sacrament. Highly susceptible to both explicit messages and implicit collective belief systems, the individual under the influence of ayahuasca is in a psychological state of heightened suggestibility. Whether the effects of the experience will ultimately be salutary or not appear in large part to be determined by the content of the explicit and implicit messages conveyed and the integrity of the religious structure.

Conclusions

It is perhaps ironic that as we prepare to transition to a new century, and a new millennium, interest in the ancient arts of transcendence has begun to increase. From first contact, some 500 years ago, the Europeans who came to the Americas scorned and demonized the psychoactive plants the indigenous peoples used in their healing practices and religious rituals. Not deemed worthy of serious investigation, plant hallucinogens such as ayahuasca remained of interest only to a handful of maverick anthropologists and ethnobotanists. Recently, however, efforts at initiating formal multidisciplinary study of ayahuasca have kindled hopes that rigorous evaluation of this Amazonian plant concoction may yield valuable new information about cross-cultural belief systems, the range of mental function and novel paradigms for healing.

From a variety of perspectives, the study of ayahuasca represents an opportunity to advance our knowledge of the human condition and the myriad conditions which influence it. Through anthropological examination of the role such plant hallucinogens have played in indigenous cultures, we may determine how particular structures and cultural contexts channel experience and optimize safety. And through the utilization of state of the art research methodologies and advanced neuroscience technologies, critical new information may become available to the fields of medicine and psychiatry. From a biological reductionistic perspective, the effects of ayahuasca on the serotonergic system in particular may lead to a new understanding of neural mechanisms responsible for central nervous system function (Callaway et al. 1994; Grob et al. 1996; McKenna et al. 1998). New models for treatment utilizing this powerful plant hallucinogen will need to incorporate knowledge gleaned both from anthropological studies of set and setting as observed within shamanic practice, as well as psychobiologic investigations of neurotransmitter and neuroendocrine effects of ayahuasca in order to achieve optimal response.

As knowledge of the highly unusual and intriguing ayahuasca experience spreads, care will have to be taken to prevent its exploitation and unsafe utilization. Already, concern has been expressed about "drug tourism" in the Amazon involving North American and European travelers in search of adventure and novel experience (Dobkin de Rios 1994). Not only do individuals often place themselves in danger through casual experimentation with unknown brews in what can be an uncontrolled and unpredictable setting, but also may have a detrimental influence upon the local cultures. And given the hyper-suggestible effects of all hallucinogens, risks may also exist when individuals allow themselves to be guided by others with questionable integrity and limited expertise. Care will also have to be taken to establish pharmacologic safety parameters for ayahuasca use, with particular attention given to potential adverse interactions with conventional pharmaceutical medications (Callaway and Grob 1998).

The study of ayahuasca represents a challenge to mainstream culture through the phenomenon of new and novel forms of religious practice, exemplified by the ayahuasca churches of Brazil which have lately spread to North America and Europe. As with the case of other plant hallucinogens employed as religious sacraments, in particular the use of peyote by the Native American Church, vital questions regarding freedom of religious practice will have to be addressed. The health professions of modernity will also need to confront the challenges of responding to the potential salutary effects of this ancient plant medicine traditionally utilized within the context of healing paradigms long regarded as alien and inconsequential. Tentative evidence of ayahuasca's capacity to facilitate healing and recuperative responses in individuals inflicted with psychiatric disorders (Grob et al. 1996) and medical illness (Topping 1998) necessitate further rigorous research investigation to establish the validity of these preliminary findings. Questions of ayahuasca's putative role in the treatment of addictive disorders, antisocial behavior or even neoplastic disease are compelling questions awaiting further exploration. To accurately determine ayahuasca's potential value as a medicine, it will ultimately be necessary to move beyond the boundaries of conventional treatment models and incorporate the lessons learned by past and distant cultures. Only then, as ancient technologies of transcendence are embedded within modern research methodologies, will we discover what true value this mysterious vine of the soul may have to us and our descendants.

References

Adovasio, J. M. & C. F. Fry. 1976. Prehistoric psychotropic drug use in northeastern Mexico and trans-Pecos Texas. *Economic Botany* 20:94–96.

Andritzky, W. 1989. Sociopsychotherapeutic functions of ayahuasca healing in Amazonia. *Journal of Psychoactive Drugs* 21:77–89.

Beringer, K. 1928. Uber ein neues, auf das extrapyramidal-motorische System wirkendes Alkaloid (Banisterin). *Nervenarztv* 1:265–75.

Bianchi, A. & G. Samorini. 1993. Plants in association with ayahuasca. *Jahrbuch für Ethnomedizin* (Yearbook of Ethnomedicine) 2:21–42.

Bravo, G. &. C. Grob. 1989. Shamans, sacraments and psychiatrists. *Journal of Psychoactive Drugs* 21:123–28.

Burroughs, W. S. & A. Ginsberg. 1963. *The Yagé Letters*. San Francisco: City Lights Books.

Callaway, J. C. 1988. A proposed mechanism for the visions of dream sleep. *Medical Hypotheses* 26:119–24.

———. 1994. Some chemistry and pharmacology of ayahuasca. *Jahrbuch für Ethnomedizin* (Yearbook of Ethnomedicine) 3:295–298.

———. 1995. DMTs in the human brain, *Jahrbuch fér Ethnomedizin* (Yearbook of Ethnomedicine) 4:45–54.

Callaway, J. C., M. M. Airaksinen, D. J. McKenna, G. S. Brito, & C. S. Grob. 1994. Platelet serotonin uptake sites increased in drinkers of ayahuasca. *Psychopharmacology* 116:385–387.

Callaway, J. C., L. P. Raymon, W. L. Hearn, D. J. McKenna, C. S. Grob, G. S. Brito, & D. C. Mash. 1996. Quantitation of *N,N*-dimethyltryptamine and harmala alkaloids in human plasma after oral dosing with ayahuasca. *Journal of Analytical Toxicology* 20:492–97.

Callaway, J. C., D. H. McKenna, C. S. Grob, G. S. Brito, L. P. Raymon, R. E. Poland, E. N. Andrade, E. O. Andrade, & D. C., Mash. 1999. Pharmacology of hoasca alkaloids in healthy humans. *Journal of Ethnopharmacology,* in press.

Callaway, J. C. & C. S. Grob. 1998. Ayahuasca preparations and serotonin reuptake inhibitors: a potential combination for severe adverse interactions. *Journal of Psychoactive Drugs* 30:367–69.

Dobkin de Rios, M. 1971. Ayahuasca, the healing vine. *International Journal of Social Psychiatry* 17:256–69.

———. 1972. *Visionary Vine: Hallucinogenic Healing in the Peruvian Amazon*. San Francisco: Chandler Publishing.

———. 1984. *Hallucinogens: Cross-Cultural Perspectives*. Albuquerque: University of New Mexico Press.

———. 1994. Drug tourism in the Amazon, *Jahrbuch für Ethnomedizin* (Yearbook of Ethnomedicine) 3:307–14.

Devereux, G. 1958. Cultural thought models in primitive and modern psychiatric theories. *Psychiatry* 21:359–74.

Dobkin de Rios, M. & C. S. Grob. 1994. Hallucinogens, suggestibility and adolescence in cross-cultural perspective. *Jahrbuch für Ethnomedizin* (Yearbook of Ethnomedicine) 3:123–32.

Eliade, M. 1964. *Shamanism: Arachaic Techniques of Ecstasy.* Princeton, NJ: Princeton University Press.

Flores, F. A. &: W. H. Lewis. 1978. Drinking the South American hallucinogen ayahuasca. *Economic Botany* 32:154–56.

Grob, C. S. 1994. Psychiatric research with hallucinogens: What have we learned? *Jahrbuch für Ethnomedizin* (Yearbook of Ethnomedicine) 3:91–112.

Grob, C. S. & M. Dobkin de Rios. 1992. Adolescent drug use in cross-cultural perspective, *Journal of Drug Issues* 22:121–38.

Grob, C. S., D. J. McKenna, J. C. Callaway, G. S. Brito, E. S. Neves, G. Oberlaender, O. L. Saide, E. Labigalini, C. Tacla, C. T. Miranda, R. J. Strassman, & K. B. Boone. 1996. Human psychopharmacology of hoasca, a plant hallucinogen used in ritual context in Brazil. *Journal of Nervous and Mental Disease* 184:86–94.

Groisman, A. & A. B. Sell. 1995. "Healing power": cultural-neurophenomenological therapy of Santo Daime. *Yearbook Cross-Cultural Medicine* 6:241–55.

Guerra, F. 1971. *The Pre-Columbian Mind.* London: Seminar Press.

Harner, M., ed. 1973a. *Hallucinogens and Shamanism.* London: Oxford University Press.

———. 1973b. Common themes in South American Indian yagé experiences. In *Hallucinogens and Shamanism,* ed. M. Harner, 155–75. London: Oxford University Press.

Huxley, A. 1977. *Moksha: Writings on Psychedelics and the Visionary Experience.* Los Angeles: J. P. Tarcher.

Kensinger, K. B. 1973. *Banisteriopsis* usage among the Peruvian Cashinuaha. In *Hallucinogens and Shamanism,* ed. M. Harner, 1–14. London: Oxford University Press.

Kusel, H. 1965. Ayahuasca drinkers among the Chama Indians of northeast Peru. *Psychedelic Review* 6:58–66.

Lewin, L. 1929. *Banisteria Caapi, ein neues Rauschgift und Heilmittel.* Berlin: Verlag von Georg Stilke.

Ludwig, A. M. 1969. Altered states of consciousness. In *Altered States of Consciousness,* ed. C. T. Tart, 11–24. New York: John Wiley and Sons.

Mabit, J. 1988. Ayahuasca Hallucinations Among Healers in the Peruvian Upper Amazon. Document de Travail. Lima: Instituto Frances de Estudios Andinos.

Mabit, J., R. Giove, & J. Vega. 1995. Takiwasi: the use of Amazonian shamanism to rehabilitate drug addicts. *Yearbook Cross-Cultural Medicine* 6:257–885.

McKenna, D. J., G. H. N. Towers, & F. S. Abbott. 1984. Monoamine oxidase inhibitors in South American hallucinogenic plants: tryptamine and beta-carboline constituents of ayahuasca. *Journal of Ethnopharmacology* 10:195–223.

McKenna, D. J., J. C. Callaway, & C. S. Grob. 1998. The scientific investigation of ayahuasca: a review of past and current research. *Heffter Review of Psychedelic Research* 1:65–77.

Naranjo, C. 1967. Psychotropic properties of the harmala alkaloids. In *Ethnopharmacologic Search for Psychoactive Drugs,* eds. D. H. Efron, R. Holmstedt, & N. S. Klein, 385–91. U. S. Public Health Service Publication No. 1645. Washington, D. C.: GPO.

———. 1973. *The Healing Journey: New Approaches to Consciousness.* New York: Random House.

Ott, J. 1993. Pharmacotheon: *Entheogenic Drugs: Their Plant Sources and History.* Kennewick, WA: Natural Products.

———. 1994a. *Ayahuasca Analogues: Pangæan Entheogens.* Kennewick, WA: Natural Products.

———. 1994b. Ayahuasca and ayahuasca analogues: pangæan entheogens for the new millennium. *Jahrbuch für Ethnomedizin* (Yearbook of Ethnomedicine) 3:285–93.

———. 1999. Pharmahuasca: human pharmacology of oral DM plus harmine. *Journal of Psychoactive Drugs,* in press.

Pennes, H. H. & P. H. Hoch. 1957. Psychotomimetics, clinical and theoretical considerations: harmine, win-2299 and nalline. *American Journal of Psychiatry* 113:887–92.

Reichel-Dolmatoff, G. 1975. *The Shaman and the Jaguar.* Philadelphia: Temple University Press.

Sanchez-Ramos, J. R. 1991. Banisterine and Parkinson's Disease. *Clinical Neuropharmacology* 14:391–402.

Schultes, R. E. & A. Hofmann. 1992. *Plants of the Gods: Their Sacred, Healing and Hallucinogenic Powers.* Rochester, VT: Healing Arts Press.

Schultes, R. E. & M. Winkelman. The principal American hallucinogenic plants and their bioactive and therapeutic properties. *Yearbook Cross-Cultural Medicine Psychotherapy* 6:205–39.

Strassman, R. J., C. R. Qualls, E. H. Uhlenhuth, & R. Kellner. 1994. Dose-response study of *N,N*-dimethyltryptamine in humans. *Archives of General Psychiatry* 51:98–108.

Taussig, M. 1987. *Shamanism, Colonialism and the Wild Man: A Study in Terror and Healing.* Chicago: University of Chicago Press.

Topping, D. M. 1998. Ayahuasca and cancer: one man's experience. *MAPS* 8(3):22–26.

Torres, C. M., D. B. Repke, & K. Chan. 1991. Snuff powders from pre-hispanic San Pedro de Atacama: chemical contextural analysis. *Current Anthropology* 32:640–49.

Turner, W. J. et al. 1955. Concerning theories of indoles in schizophrenigenesis. *American Journal of Psychiatry* 112:466–67.

Villavicencio, M. 1858. *Geografía de la República del Ecuador.* New York: R. Craigshead.

Wasson, R. G., S. Kramrisch, J. Ott, & C. A. P. Ruck. 1986. *Persephone's Quest: Entheogens and the Origins of Religion.* New Haven, CT: Yale University Press.

Appendix B

Deconstructing Ecstasy: The Politics of MDMA Research

Charles S. Grob, M.D.

WHAT IS *Ecstasy?* Defined by the *New Webster's Dictionary* as a state of intense overpowering emotion, a condition of exultation or mental rapture induced by beauty, music, artistic creation or the contemplation of the divine, ecstasy derives etymologically from the ancient Greek *ekstasis,* which means flight of the soul from the body. The anthropologist, Mircea Eliade, who explored the roots of religious experience in his book *Shamanism: Archaic Techniques of Ecstasy,* has described the function of this intense state of mind among aboriginal peoples. Select individuals are called to become shamans, a role specializing in inducing ecstatic states of trance where the soul is believed to leave the body and ascend to the sky or descend to the underworld. The shaman is thus considered a "technician of the sacred," having been initiated through a process of isolation, ritual solitude, suffering and the imminence of death. Such initiation into the function of ecstatic states of consciousness, always accompanied by comprehensive tutelage from tribal elders, allows the shaman to assume for his tribal group the vital role of intermediary, or conduit, between the profane world of everyday existence and the sacred domains of alternative reality (Eliade, 1951; Schultes and Hofmann, 1992).

Modern conceptualizations of ecstasy, however, have expanded far beyond the realm of scholarly inquiry on archaic religions to the reach of contemporary cultural politics and scientific inquiry. As a cultural commodity, ecstasy has become emblematic of a social movement attracting increasing numbers of disaffected youth in Europe and North America. Meeting together in the hundreds and the thousands, large groups of young people have congregated to engage in collective *trance dances,* or *raves,* often fueled by the ingestion of a synthetic psychoactive substance, known as *Ecstasy.* Arousing apprehension among parents and civic authorities, perplexed by this changing pattern of behavior among youth, the phenomenon of *ecstasy* culture has riveted societal concern on the potential dangers of its increasingly notorious chemical sacrament. In spite of substantial media coverage, along with millions of federal dollars for basic science research on neural mechanisms for possible brain injury caused by *Ecstasy,* however, full understanding of both its medical consequences and cultural impact have remained elusive.

Even within the current social context of harsh Drug War era legal penalties, *Ecstasy* use has climbed sharply among young people. A vast and unanticipated social experiment has occurred, with millions of adolescents and young adults worldwide consuming a drug which has eluded definitive understanding and over which societal and medical controversies persist. Given the magnitude of public health and cultural implications, an open and comprehensive review of the existing state of knowledge, from diverse perspectives, needs to be pursued. The outcome of such an inquiry into this modern rendering of the archaic technique of ecstasy should facilitate a more effective and salutary understanding and response to the condition Euro-American medicine and culture currently confront.

Social History

Since the early 1980s, the drug *Ecstasy* has commonly been considered to be 3,4-methylenedioxymethamphetamine (MDMA), though this identification has become increasingly problematic over the last decade. Classified as a phenethylamine, MDMA chemically has been noted to have structural similarities to both amphetamine and the hallucinogen, mescaline, as well as the essential oil safrole, found in sassafras and nutmeg. Though patented by Merck Pharmaceuticals in Germany prior to the First World War, MDMA was not explored in animal models until the 1950s, when the U.S. Army Intelligence undertook the serial investigation of a variety of psychoactive compounds with potential "brain washing" application. MDMA itself was never administered to humans during this Cold War–inspired phase of investigation, and remained unexplored until the 1970s. Its more hallucinogenic and longer acting analogue, 3,4-methylenedioxyamphetamine (MDA), however, was the object of official investigation as part of the infamous MK-ULTRA program of the fifties and sixties and had been administered to Army "volunteers," including one who was inadvertently overdosed and killed. Initial scientific investigations of MDMA itself occurred during the 1970s following the termination of military involvement, and were conducted by university- and industry-based medicinal chemists. Researchers, extending their inquiries to the effects on humans, were enthusiastic over the drug's unique psychoactive profile. The development of a new class of centrally active compounds was proposed, one with suggested therapeutic capacities, which would be named Entactogens, after a salient psychological feature of the drug, its capacity "to touch within." (Shulgin, 1986; Shulgin, 1990; Shulgin and Nichols, 1978; Shulgin and Shulgin, 1991).

Early scientific investigators, though without formal psychological schooling, were struck by MDMA's capacity to help people open up and talk honestly about themselves and their relationships, without defensive conditioning intervening. For several hours anxiety and fear appeared to melt away, even in subjects who were chronically constricted and apprehensive. By the late 1970s, a small number of mental health professionals had been introduced to the drug's range of psychoactive effects. Particularly impressed by MDMA's capacity to induce profound states of empathy, one of the strongest predictors of positive psychotherapeutic outcome, these first psychologists and psychiatrists who encountered the drug believed they had come across a valuable new treatment. First called *Adam,* to signify "the condition of primal innocence and unity with all life," MDMA-augmented therapy functioned by reducing defensive barriers, while enhancing communication and intimacy. Hailed as a "penicillin for the soul," MDMA was said to be useful in treating a wide range of conditions, including post-traumatic stress, phobias, psychosomatic disorders, depression, suicidality, drug addiction, relationship difficulties and the psychological distress of terminal illness (Adamson, 1985; Adamson and Metzner, 1988; Grinspoon and Bakalar, 1986; Greer and Tolbert, 1986; Downing, 1986; Riedlinger and Riedlinger, 1994).

Conscious of the lessons of history from the 1950s to the early 1970s, when researchers had been prevented from continuing their promising investigations of hallucinogen treatment models because of the cultural reaction to their spread among young people, efforts were initially undertaken to restrict the flow of information on MDMA. Hoping to avoid the fate of LSD and maintain MDMA's still legal status, its use for several years remained limited to a relatively small group of pharmacologists and health professionals. MDMA's advantages over the better-known hallucinogens as a putative psychotherapeutic adjunct were also noted. Compared to LSD, the prototype hallucinogen of the twentieth century, MDMA was a relatively mild, short-acting drug capable of facilitating heightened states of introspection and intimacy along with temporary freedom from anxiety and depression, yet without distracting alterations in perception, body image and sense of self. MDMA had neither the pharmacologic profile nor the provocative reputation of LSD and, so they hoped, would not suffer the fate of political reaction and legal censure as the hallucinogens had in the late 1960s (Grof, 1990; Bakalar and Grinspoon, 1990; Grob, 1998).

It proved difficult, however, to keep MDMA a secret. Catalyzed by the call for hearings challenging the proposed scheduling of MDMA by the DEA, sensationalized media reports about a new psychotherapeutic "miracle medicine" began to attract the interest of drug dealers suddenly aware of the large potential profits to be made selling MDMA to young people.

Soon, MDMA began to emerge as an alternative recreational drug on some college campuses, particularly in California and Texas, where for a period of time MDMA replaced cocaine as a new drug of choice. Although still popular as *Adam* among psychotherapists, MDMA now acquired a new name among youth, *Ecstasy*. In point of fact, the transformation of *Adam* into *Ecstasy* appears to have been a marketing decision reached by an enterprising distributor searching for an alternative code name, who concluded that it would not be profitable to take advantage of the drug's most salient features. "*Ecstasy* was chosen for obvious reasons," this individual later reported, "because it would sell better than calling it *Empathy*. *Empathy* would be more appropriate, but how many people know what it means?" (Eisner, 1989; Beck and Rosenbaum, 1994).

The days of MDMA being the singular tool among an underground of informed psychotherapists were over. Now popularly known as *Ecstasy*, MDMA had been appropriated by the youth culture for use as a recreational drug. Spurred by media accounts reporting on both its suggested role in treatment and its new reputation as a "fun drug" among the young, use of MDMA spread. By the mid-1980s the inevitable political response began to take form. With the clear intention of tightening the federal regulatory controls of what was still a legal drug, the U.S. Drug Enforcement Administration (DEA) invoked the Emergency Scheduling Act and convened formal hearings in 1985 to determine the fate of MDMA. These highly publicized hearings, however, achieved the unintended effect of further raising public awareness of the new *Ecstasy* phenomenon, and led to marked increases in manufacturing and marketing of the drug. Media accounts polarized opinion, pitting enthusiastic claims of MDMA by proponents on the one hand, versus dire warnings of unknown dangers to the nation's youth on the other. Coverage of the MDMA scheduling controversy included a national daytime television talk show (the Phil Donahue program) highlighting the surprise disclosure by a prominent University of Chicago neuroscientist that recent (but as yet unpublished) research had detected "brain damage" in rats injected with large quantities of MDA (3,4-Methylenedioxyamphetamine), an analogue and metabolite of MDMA.

Public debate was further confounded by the frequent confusion of MDMA with MPTP (1-Methyl-4-phenyl-1,2,3,6-tetrahydropyridine), a dopaminergic neurotoxin that had recently been shown to have induced severe Parkinson's-like disorders in opiate addicts using a new synthetic heroin substitute. With growing concerns over the dangers of new "designer drugs," public discussion took an increasingly discordant tone (Beck and Morgan, 1986).

In the spring of 1985, a series of scheduling hearings on MDMA were conducted by the DEA in several U.S. cites where a collective of physicians, psychologists, researchers and lawyers gave testimony that MDMA's healing potential should not be lost to the therapeutic community. After hearing the dueling sentiments expressed by federal regulators and by those opposed to controls, the DEA administrative law judge presiding over the hearings determined on the weight of the evidence presented that there was in fact sufficient indication for the safe utilization of MDMA under medical supervision and recommended Schedule III status. Not obliged to follow the recommendations of his administrative law judge, however, and expressing grave concerns that MDMA's growing abuse liability posed a serious threat to public health and safety, the DEA director overruled the advisement and ordered that MDMA be placed in the most restrictive category, Schedule I. Since then, with the exception of a three-month period in late 1987 and early 1988 when it was briefly unscheduled due to a court challenge, MDMA has remained classified as a Schedule I substance (Young, 1986; Lawn, 1986).

In the decade following the MDMA scheduling controversy, patterns of use experienced a marked shift. With the failure to establish official sanction for MDMA treatment, most psychotherapists who had used the drug adjunctively in their work ceased to do so, unwilling to violate the law and jeopardize their livelihood through the use of a now illegal drug. In the wake of the highly publicized scheduling hearings, however, use among young people escalated. By the late 1980s interest in *Ecstasy* had spread from the United States across the Atlantic to Europe, where it became the drug of choice at marathon dance parties called *raves*. Beginning on the

Spanish island of Ibiza, spreading across the Continent, and then back to the United States, *Ecstasy*-catalyzed *raves* drew increasingly large numbers of young people, often attracting more than 10,000 participants to a single event. Although use in the United States has tended to be cyclical, waxing and waning depending upon an often erratic supply, popularity in Europe remained high through the 1990s. With multiple illicit laboratories, including pharmaceutical manufacturers in former *Iron Curtain* countries, the European youth recreational drug market has been saturated with *Ecstasy* over the past decade (Saunders, 1993; Saunders, 1995; Capdevila, 1995).

By the late 1980s, the *Ecstasy* scene had attained particular prominence among young people in the United Kingdom. Between 1990 and 1995, British authorities estimated that the use of *Ecstasy* increased by over 4,000 percent. Starting in small London dance clubs, word rapidly spread of the euphoric, mood-altering properties induced by *Ecstasy,* leading to larger and larger events throughout the British Isles. Almost overnight an enormous black market for *Ecstasy* was created. Leisure patterns among the young began to change, with *Ecstasy* to an increasing degree replacing alcohol as a generational drug of choice. By the early 1990s, the economic and social certainties of the past in Great Britain had started to change. The free market boom pursued throughout the eighties by the Thatcher government had ended in recession, with increasing unemployment and constricting opportunities, particularly for young people. The freeing of inhibitions, the peer bonding and the sense of community engendered by *Ecstasy*'s dance floor pharmacology provided a release from the oppressive social atmosphere and a sense that "all could be made right in the world." The *Ecstasy* scene had become, in the eyes of many observers, the largest youth cultural phenomenon that Great Britain had ever seen (Collin, 1998).

With the rapid expansion of *Ecstasy* culture in the United Kingdom, criminal gangs began to sense the opportunity for amassing large profits and moved in on the developing drug scene, rapidly taking control of the manufacturing and marketing of *Ecstasy*. Motivated solely by financial return and disinterested in the "purity" of the phenomenon, the quality of distributed *Ecstasy* began to erode. Other drugs began to replace MDMA as the sole component of *Ecstasy* pills, including diverse phenethylamine analogues (e.g. MDA, MDE), amphetamines, cocaine, opiates and even the dissociative anesthetic ketamine. The increasing use of methamphetamine, sold both openly and as adulterated *Ecstasy*, began to change *rave* culture from a context of communal celebration to one of aggressive euphoria. Ignorance and lack of available information also pervaded the youth *Ecstasy* scene, as dangerous degrees of polydrug use increasingly became the norm. Intent to "prolong the buzz," users began to "stack" multiple doses of *Ecstasy*, along with alcohol and whatever other drugs were available. In just a few years, the *Ecstasy* scene had drifted far from what its earliest proponents had extolled as the gentle opening and spiritual nature of MDMA to the faster paced, increasingly dangerous, anything-goes polydrug context of the evolving dance drug industry (Ziporyn, 1986; Buchanan and Brown, 1988; Wolff *et al.*, 1996; Winstock and King, 1996; Furnari *et al.*, 1998).

Although various estimates have been given on the extent of current *Ecstasy* use in the United States and Western Europe, the exact incidence is not known. Saunders has stated that "millions" of young people in the United Kingdom have taken *Ecstasy*. A Harris Opinion Poll for the BBC in Great Britain presented data that 31% of people between the ages of 16 and 25 admitted to taking *Ecstasy*, most often at dance clubs, and that 67% reported that their friends had tried the drug. In a survey of school children across the whole of England, 4.25% of 14-year-olds and, in another survey 6.0% of those aged 14 and 15 were reported to have taken *Ecstasy*. More recently, 13% of British university students questioned about their drug histories admitted to having tried *Ecstasy*. The popular British press has reported that an estimated 500,000–1,000,000 young people in Great Britain take *Ecstasy* every weekend (Harris, 1982; Beck, 1993; Sylvester, 1995; Sharkey, 1996; Saunders and Doblin, 1996; Parrott, 1998).

In the United States, according to a 1993 National Institute on Drug Abuse survey, 2% of all United States college students had admitted to taking *Ecstasy* in the previous 12 months. By the end of the decade, 8% of high school seniors reported having tried *Ecstasy.* A well-publicized 1987 interview study of Stanford University undergraduate students reported that 39% had taken *Ecstasy* at least once in their lives. Later controversy revealed, however, that the research design was flawed by using data collected at the Stanford Student Union on Friday and Saturday nights where attractive young research assistants would solicit information from students. A methodologically stronger survey at Tulane University found that 24% of over 1,200 students questioned had experimented with *Ecstasy.* By the early 1990s, *Ecstasy* was described as having the greatest growth potential among all illicit drugs in the United States, with tens of thousands of new users allegedly introduced to the drug every month, particularly within the context of the *rave* scene. (Peroutka, 1987; NIDA, 1993; NIDA, 1999; Newmeyer, 1993; Cuomo *et al.,* 1994; D. J. McKenna, pers. com.).

As *Ecstasy* culture continued to grow in the nineties, youthful adherents were deprived of accurate information about the chemical catalysts they were ingesting. From inadequately informed media and chains of improbable rumor, a number of myths remained in general circulation among young ravers, ranging from beliefs that their coveted drug of choice was entirely safe to other convictions that *Ecstasy* could induce horrific nervous system damage, including the draining of spinal fluid. While media trumpeted sensationalist accounts of *The Agony of Ecstasy,* a lack of clarity and understanding of the drug's true effects pervaded the youth scene. The knowledge accrued during the period of underground psychotherapy in the late 1970s and early 1980s that with repeated use MDMA's positive effects attenuated and negative side effects accentuated (thus making it the ideal therapeutic agent, to be used sparingly and with minimal abuse potential) had not filtered through to the young denizens of the burgeoning *Ecstasy* culture. Coupled with the omnipotence of youth, this ignorance of the drug's basic psychopharmacology led to wide scale over-use of the drug. As participants returned to weekend dance parties repeatedly from week to week, the prolonged use of *Ecstasy* began to take its toll. Over time and repeated use, the euphoria and the empathy would lessen, to be replaced by a jittery amphetamine-like experience. For days after their night of *Ecstasy* it was not uncommon for *ravers,* particularly those with some underlying vulnerability, to report dysphoric mood and cognitive dulling. Although *Ecstasy* was not physically addictive, certain individuals would demonstrate clear patterns of psychologically compulsive behavior. A *macho ingestion syndrome* typified some young men with a proclivity for ingesting five or more doses at a single setting. Safety limits that had been appreciated by older investigators from a long ago era hoping to develop new tools for healing no longer appeared to be operative in this new postmodern world of youth recreational drug culture.

The preferred mode of *Ecstasy* experience, the dance club setting, also appeared to heighten the risks for young *ravers*. Gathered closely together in crowded environments, often with poor ventilation and high ambient temperatures, large numbers of young people would dance exuberantly late into the night. By the early-1990s, reports of individuals dying of heat stroke during *raves* began to surface. Though relatively small in number compared to the enormous degree of use among youth in the United Kingdom, around 15 fatalities per year have been reported. In each of these cases, *Ecstasy* ingestion was associated with a catastrophic hyperthermic reaction leading to disseminated intravascular coagulation (DIC), rhabdomyolysis, and acute renal and hepatic failure, culminating in death. In contrast to the long forgotten therapeutic model of relaxing in a peaceful setting with easy access to sufficient fluid replacement, many of these tragic events occurred in dance clubs where management restricted supplies of water in order to increase the sales of soft drinks. In one particularly unscrupulous establishment, the water taps were reportedly turned off in the bathrooms while tap water was sold over the counter at the bar for the price of a beer (Henry *et al.*, 1992; Matthews and Jones, 1992; Randall, 1992).

As awareness grew that *Ecstasy* could under certain circumstances cause injury to users, a movement arose within the *rave* community to ensure greater protection from dangerous influences. Efforts to promote harm-reduction practices at *Ecstasy*-fueled dances, however, were solely supported by the community and their adherents. Virtually all government and enforcement agencies, by contrast, have appeared to interpret the harm-reduction process entirely through the eyes of legal censure and prohibition. Privately sponsored safe dancing campaigns developed a code of conduct for *raves,* attempting to minimize the degree of risk encountered by young *ravers.* These harm reduction efforts would emphasize the monitoring of air quality and ambient temperature, provision of *chill out* rooms, easy access to cold water taps and the distribution of drug risk information.

Another ominous development of *Ecstasy* culture was the growing awareness that to an increasing degree not all *Ecstasy* was MDMA. Over a relatively short period of time, the shift to clandestine large-scale criminal manufacture and distribution networks had led to a breakdown of quality control. Adulterated black market *Ecstasy* flowed freely through the youth culture. *Ecstasy* could be MDMA (often of low quality), or it could be any one of a variety of other drugs. By the mid-nineties, only an estimated 40% of *Ecstasy* was actually MDMA. Some of this *ersatz Ecstasy* proved to be relatively innocuous, and included aspirin, caffeine and low dosages of ephedrine. Other batches proved to be far more hazardous, however, including the emergence at the end of the decade on both sides of the Atlantic of large quantities of dextromethorphan, a cough suppressant with powerful dissociative properties at higher dosages. Sold as *Ecstasy,* dextromethorphan could induce an overwhelming and prolonged experience. Particularly within the context of a *rave,* dextromethorphan was increasingly recognized as a highly dangerous substance, capable of causing serious medical harm both when taken alone and when taken in combination with MDMA. Besides competing with MDMA for cytochrome p450 2D6 hepatic enzymes, and thus impeding MDMA's metabolism and elimination, dextromethorphan's anticholinergic effects also blocked perspiration, increasing the risk of dangerous overheating. To counter this insidious threat to the health and safety of young *dance* culture aficionados, harm reduction efforts have recently been directed towards providing on-site and affordable qualitative laboratory analyses of *Ecstasy* samples (Shewan *et al.*, 1996; Doblin, 1996; King, 1998; Schifano *et al.*, 1998; Sferios, 1999).

Loathe to be perceived as providing any tacit validation of the *Ecstasy* culture movement, government and health institutions have shunned the harm reduction approach, instead relying upon the message of primary prevention. Young people should simply avoid taking *Ecstasy,* they should *just say no!* To reinforce this zero tolerance strategy, considerable outlays of funding have been directed at establishing the precise mechanisms of destructive action of the drug. The study of MDMA neurotoxicity has received millions of dollars of government research funding over the last decade and a half to elaborate the magnitude of functional and structural injury to animal neurotransmitter systems. Experimentation using human subjects has in contrast received far less support, with none provided for efforts intended to explore the long-neglected MDMA treatment paradigms. While retrospective studies of human *Ecstasy* users have fit nicely into the prevailing belief system that MDMA may cause serious brain injury, it has proved virtually impossible to conduct any investigation of its putative healing capacity. Though never disproven, the MDMA treatment model has never been given the opportunity to test its safety and efficacy in alleviating suffering under ideal controlled circumstances. Efforts to initiate treatment studies on refractory patient populations in the United States have to date not been successful in obtaining final approval from federal regulatory agencies (although the FDA has recently expressed a willingness to approve well-designed treatment studies in refractory patient populations). Three basic Phase 1 prospective studies of normal human volunteers to study psychological effects, physiologic response, pharmacokinetics and neurotransmitter mechanisms have been allowed that administered pure MDMA in hospital research settings in the United States (at Harbor-UCLA Medical Center, the University of California San Francisco School of Medicine and the Wayne State University School of Medicine) (Grob *et al.*, 1996; Tancer and Schuster, 1997; Tancer and Johanson, 1999; Harris *et al.*, 1999). By contrast, attempts extending from the mid-1980s to the present to use MDMA in controlled treatment protocols have not as yet received approval.

Only in Europe, in Switzerland from 1988 to 1993, were a group of clinical psychiatrists granted permission from their government to treat their patients with MDMA. Although authorities had failed to insist upon the implementation of prospective research designs, a retrospective analysis of treatment outcomes was eventually conducted (Gasser, 1995a; Gasser, 1995b). That study examined MDMA-augmented psychotherapy of 121 patients, providing very encouraging results, indicating high degrees of treatment response along with acceptable safety parameters. In spite of those conclusions, subsequent and better designed investigations have not been conducted. Elsewhere throughout the world there have been only two other MDMA treatment protocols which have been submitted to their respective regulatory authorities. One is a study of rape victims with post-traumatic stress disorder at the Universitat Autonoma de Madrid in Spain. The other is a proposed investigation at the Harbor-UCLA Medical Center in the United States of patients with end-stage cancer whose depression, anxiety, alienation and pain have not responded to conventional therapies. A variety of plausible explanations for the failure to initiate formal programs of MDMA treatment research could be suggested, ranging from the need to maintain a political distance from illicit *Ecstasy* use to the long-entrenched aversion to associating with the old hallucinogen treatment model. The central obstacle to formal regulatory approval, however, has remained the ongoing focus on the possibility that MDMA causes brain damage. Whether pure MDMA will ever be permitted in an optimally controlled treatment research context might ultimately hinge on the question of neurotoxicity.

Neurotoxicity

Pharmacologically, MDMA's site of action is largely within the serotonergic neurotransmitter system. Serotonin (5-hydroxytryptamine, 5-HT) is one of the monoamine neurotransmitters of the brain, and is synthesized from tryptophan through the intermediate compound 5-hydroxytryptophan. Serotonin is synthesized within 5-HT neurons, and is stored in synaptic vesicles. It is released by these vesicles into the synaptic cleft in response to the firing of 5-HT neurons, exerts an effect upon both pre- and post-synaptic receptor sites, and is then taken back up into the 5-HT neuron where it is again stored in synaptic vesicles. The serotonin neurotransmitter system is believed to play a critical role in the regulation of mood, anxiety, sleep, appetite, aggression, sexuality and temperature regulation.

The field of amphetamine analogue neurotoxicity began in the early

1960s, with the discovery that particular drugs were capable of causing severe changes within different neurotransmitter systems. Disruptions of the serotonergic (5-HT) system was first observed to occur in animal models injected with what would become known as the prototype serotonin neurotoxin, para-chloroamphetamine (PCA) (Pletscher *et al.*, 1963). PCA was observed to cause a prolonged decrease in brain concentrations of serotonin and 5-hydroxyindole acetic acid (5-HIAA), the primary metabolite of serotonin, without altering norepineprine or dopamine concentrations. Later studies found that tryptophan hydroxylase (TPH), the rate limiting enzyme in serotonin biosynthesis, was markedly decreased for up to several months following PCA administration (Sanders-Bush *et al.*, 1975).

Since the mid-1980s, evidence has accumulated that MDMA is capable of inflicting major changes on the brain serotonin system in laboratory animals (McKenna and Peroutka, 1990). Preclinical studies have consistently demonstrated that MDMA induces an acute, but reversible, depletion of serotonin. These findings have included time limited but sustained lower levels of serotonin, decreased metabolite (5-HIAA) levels, loss of synthetic enzyme activity (TPH), loss of serotonin uptake and loss of uptake sites for serotonin. Unlike the far more toxic PCA, however, which has been demonstrated in animals to damage serotonergic cell bodies (Harvey *et al.*, 1975), MDMA's effects are limited to axonal projections, with evident sparing of cell bodies. Over time following exposure to repeated, high dose MDMA administration, regeneration of serotonin axons does occur, with a gradual yet measurable increase in axon density (Molliver *et al.*, 1990). Rate of recovery varies depending upon species studied, with rats demonstrating greater degrees of reversible depletion than monkeys.

The impact on serotonin systems in laboratory animals subjected to administration of MDMA has been divided into short- and long-term effects. Some of the acute effects of MDMA, including the rapid release of intracellular stores of serotonin, are believed to mediate the psychological and behavioral profile observed in humans in the first three to four hours after drug administration, whereas in animals the presumed neurotoxic effects begin to manifest about 12–24 hours later. Consequently, it is believed that neurotoxicity is not inextricably linked to the acute effects of the drug. Further demonstrating the separation between behavioral and laboratory neurotoxicity profiles has been the observation that administration to animals of fluoxetine (a serotonin re-uptake blocker) up to six hours after MDMA injection, blocks or attenuates the development of neurotoxicity (Hekmatpanah and Peroutka, 1990), whereas in human subjects the acute effects of MDMA (psychological, neuroendocrine and temperature) occur within minutes and peak in a few hours (Grob *et al.*, 1996).

Most animal investigations of MDMA have revolved around establishing the extent of and mechanisms underlying neurotoxicity. Rats administered multiple high dosages of MDMA undergo what are described as serotonergic neurotoxic changes which persist for many months before full neurochemical recovery occurs. Significant variation can occur, however, with dosage, route of administration and species. An important area of neurotoxicity research has been the histopathological study of brain sections of animals given substantial dosages of MDMA. This model was elaborated in the early 1980s at the University of Chicago by senior neuroscientists C. R. Schuster and Lewis Seiden, and their student, George Ricaurte. Their first major contribution to the MDMA literature was a 1985 (Ricaurte *et al.*) study of what they described as classic signs of serotonin neurotoxicity in rats injected subcutaneously twice daily for four consecutive days with 20mg/kg of the longer lasting MDMA analogue, MDA. Coincident in time with the legal MDMA hearings being conducted by the DEA, the release of the University of Chicago findings accentuated the growing fears stirred by the new and only recently publicized reports of *Ecstasy* use. The introduction of the concept of serotonin neurotoxicity into the debate over MDMA's legal status has had a lasting influence on public and scientific appraisal of the problem.

Utilizing the repeated high dose MDMA administration model in most animal experiments, investigators have found sustained effects on various aspects of serotonin neuronal architecture, specifically the axonal projections. In virtually all immunohistochemical studies, the changes induced by MDMA are limited to the axons, with evident sparing of the cell bodies. Effects also appear to be contained within the smaller distal axonal projections, and not the larger more proximal axons. Resprouting and re-generation of serotonin axon terminals does occur, although the time course for full recovery may be extensive and varies significantly between different species. The question of whether the axonal reconnections ob-served during recovery are "normal" or are damaged, however, has not as yet been definitively answered. In squirrel monkeys administered MDMA (5 mg/kg, subcutaneous) twice daily for four consecutive days, profound reductions of brain serotonin, 5-hydroxyindole acetic acid, and serotonin uptake sites persist even at 18 months (Ali *et al.*, 1993). Interestingly, the thalamus shows full recovery, while the hypothalamus shows an (apparent) overshoot in regeneration, suggesting that under some circumstances ad-ministration of MDMA can lead to a lasting reorganization of ascending serotonin projections. In a study with more relevance to the single time or occasional use, low-dose therapeutic model, a "no-effect" level in monkeys of 2.5 mg/kg MDMA administered orally every two weeks for four months (totaling eight times) was established by Ricaurte (Karel, 1994). Either be-cause of the highly politicized nature of the MDMA neurotoxicity debate, or for reasons that have as yet not been made entirely clear, this infor-mation has to date never been published in the mainstream scientific literature.

At the center of the controversy over the central nervous system effects of MDMA has been researcher George Ricaurte, who while still a student was the lead author of the 1985 paper on MDA neurotoxicity that played such a pivotal role in the DEA scheduling decision. For the following fif-teen years, first at Stanford Medical School and then at Johns Hopkins-Bayview Medical Center, Ricaurte has built one of the most influential and well-funded MDMA neurotoxicity research programs. Reluctant to support investigations designed to study MDMA's therapeutic efficacy and safety, Ricaurte has steadfastly contended that "even one dose of MDMA can lead to permanent brain damage" in humans. With each new study from his laboratory being widely publicized in the media, Ricaurte has had an instrumental role in the evolution of scientific and cultural attitudes toward MDMA. A careful examination, however, of the neurotoxicity controversy, including some of Ricaurte's key research designs and patterns of data interpretation, may lead to a clearer and more objective understanding of MDMA's full range of effects and potential to cause harm.

Investigators tracking the histopathologic changes induced by MDMA have noted substantial variability between different species' susceptibility to the phenomenon. Larger species, particularly monkey models, appeared to have far more sensitivity to the drug's neurochemical effects, and even at relatively low doses sustain persistent measurable effects (Slikker *et al.*, 1988). Compared to smaller species, including the mouse, which appeared to be far more resistant to MDMA's effects (Battaglia *et al.*, 1988; Peroutka, 1988), prolonged changes in the density of distal axon projections as seen with immunohistochemical staining were consistently observed. Given such findings, Ricaurte has given prominence to the theory of interspecies scaling (Chappell and Mordenti, 1991), which proposes that different animal groups will respond to drug effects only according to their relative size. Depending upon weight (mg/kg) and surface area (mg/m^2), different species, depending upon how large they are, will have greater or lesser susceptibility to MDMA's presumed neurotoxic effects. This argument, heavily relied upon by Ricaurte, however, is flawed in its neglect of interspecies differences in pharmacokinetics and drug metabolism.

Although animal pharmacokinetics studies have not been avidly pursued, most likely a reflection of the pharmaceutical industries' lack of interest in MDMA, a related drug, fenfluramine, has had cross-species investigations of differences in drug metabolism (Caccia *et al.*, 1982). An appetite suppressant marketed widely for years, fenfluramine was recently the subject of controversy over suggested adverse cardiac valve effects that led to its removal from the market in 1997. Although the risk of cardiac valve injury now appears to be far less than feared when the original report was published (Burger *et al.*, 1999; Schiller, 1999), the ban on the drug is not likely to be lifted any time soon, given the long-term impact of the early media reports. Interestingly, fenfluramine has also been known for years to have virtually identical long-term effects as MDMA on serotonin neurochemistry and neuronal architecture, and has similarly been the object of interest by the Ricaurte neurotoxicity team (McCann *et al.*, 1994; McCann and Ricaurte, 1995). Although the threat of fenfluramine neurotoxicity risk was used to combat industry efforts to have its isomer D-fenfluramine released on the market in the mid-1990s, the FDA approved the drug for clinical use. A critical reason behind the decision was the fact that fenfluramine had a long history of general use as an appetite suppressant, having been taken by over 25,000,000 people worldwide for more than three decades (Derome-Tremblay and Nathan, 1989), and yet no clinical syndrome of fenfluramine neurotoxicity had ever been described.

The relevance of the fenfluramine example also extends to the issue of drug metabolism. Basic pharmacokinetic studies have established that size may not necessarily be the critical determinant in species susceptibility to the immunohistochemical effect described as serotonin neurotoxicity. It is well known that there are large species differences in the pharmacokinetics and metabolism of fenfluramine (Marchant *et al.*, 1992). Interestingly, humans metabolize fenfluramine much differently than do squirrel monkeys, and are actually far closer in pharmacokinetic profile to smaller species like the rat. Humans also deaminate the drug more extensively than other species to polar inactive compounds that are excreted in the urine as conjugates. Thus, the norfenfluramine/fenfluramine metabolite ratio is much higher in most other species, particularly in the non-human primates where the level of the metabolite is 40 times greater than in humans (Johnson and Nichols, 1990; Caccia *et al.*, 1993). If fenfluramine's primary metabolite norfenfluramine has greater neurotoxicity than fenfluramine, paralleling the relationship between MDMA and its metabolite MDA, then perhaps humans have less reason to fear MDMA neurotoxicity than the Ricaurte monkey studies appear to suggest. To the degree that MDMA is as close to fenfluramine in its pharmacokinetics as it is in its serotonergic neurochemistry, then the relevance of neurotoxicity to the human example is diminished proportionally.

Nevertheless, a cavalier attitude towards MDMA's risks would be ill-advised. A variety of serious adverse events, entirely apart from the neurotoxicity hypothesis, may potentially occur. Pioneering human pharmacokinetics research with MDMA, which was recently conducted by investigators at the Institut Municipal d'Investigacio Medica and Universitat Autonoma de Barcelona, Spain, and also in the United States at the University of California San Francisco, sheds new light on the importance of safety parameters to understanding differential drug metabolism (Harris *et al.,* 1999; Mas *et al.,* 1999). In humans, various organs, particularly the cardiovascular system, experience a non-linear pharmacodynamic response to increased dosages of MDMA. With increasing dose, a disproportionate elevation of plasma levels occurs that is significantly greater than that which would have been expected from linear kinetics. From the public health and safety perspective, therefore, it would appear that a persistent fixation on the relative risks and implications of the serotonin neurotoxicity threat has hampered efforts to investigate more clinically relevant concerns, including risks of cardiac arrhythmias, hypertension, cerebrovascular accidents and adverse drug-drug interactions at higher dosage levels of MDMA (Dowling *et al.,* 1987; Manchanda and Connolly, 1993; Harrington *et al.,* 1999).

Controversy has also existed over whether MDMA (and fenfluramine) fit the precise definition of neurotoxins. Concerned that the term "neurotoxicity" has been too broadly applied, James O'Callaghan, a neurotoxicologist for the U.S. Centers for Disease Control and Prevention, has questioned many of the assumptions upon which this area of research has rested, particularly whether MDMA causes degenerative conditions of the central nervous system. O'Callaghan has demonstrated that the standard techniques used to identify classic evidence of neuronal destruction, such as astrogliosis and silver degeneration staining, do not occur in rats treated with MDMA. Disputing the use of immunohistochemical evidence to interpret the significance of long-term reorganization of brain serotonergic neurotransmitter systems, O'Callaghan takes issue with the assertion that MDMA causes classic neurotoxicity. Evidence of lowered indices of serotonin, he states, should not necessarily be equated with the destruction of serotonin axons, as one would expect in bona fide serotonin neurotoxicity, because assessments of serotonin are only indicative of the presence of this transmitter in neurons, not the actual neuronal structures themselves. In other words, O'Callaghan contends that MDMA can decrease the level of serotonin without necessarily destroying serotonergic axons, much as water could be drained from a pipe without there necessarily being structural damage to the pipe itself. Furthermore, the expected evidence of structural damage to serotonin neurons, glial proliferation, does not reliably occur. Known neurotoxins, including bilirubin, cadmium, tri-methyl tin, the dopamanergic neurotoxin MPTP and the classic serotonergic neurotoxins para-chloroamphetamine (PCA) and 5,7-dihydroxytryptamine (5,7-DHT) predictably induce a proliferation of enlarged astroglial cells. According to O'Callaghan, the failure to detect evidence of a reliable astrogliosis response caused by MDMA or fenfluramine through standard laboratory testing in rats, even in the presence of decreased neurochemical markers of serotonin, further detracts from the neurotoxicity argument and instead calls for the alternative model of "neuromodulation," where protein synthesis inhibition occurs as a natural extension of the pharmacological activity of the compounds (O'Callaghan, 1993; O'Callaghan, 1995; O'Callaghan and Miller, 1993; O'Callaghan and Miller, 1994). Of course, O'Callaghan's arguments are qualified by the relative persistence of the serotonergic deficits caused by MDMA. Simple adaptation or neuromodulation would not be expected to last for years or even months as a consequence of the application of a compound that did not in fact produce some degree of prolonged structural change. Nevertheless, the functional significance of such changes remains unclear.

Debate over the clinical relevance of the MDMA neurotoxicity data, along with the political pressures of the time, have restricted the development of alternative perspectives and interpretations of serotonergic system change. Examining the implications of extensive serotonin neurotoxicity induced by administration of the classic serotonin neurotoxin, 5,7-dihydroxytryptamine (5,7-DHT), neuroscientist Efrain Azmitia of the New York University School of Medicine has raised the question of brain plasticity. Using basic laboratory models, Azmitia has explored the possibility that serotonin may actually function as a neurodevelopmental signal. Through damage to specific populations of serotonergic neurons in the adult brain, latent mechanisms for new growth and axonal sprouting are reactivated and a compensatory growth response occurs from neighboring undamaged neurons. The implications of this *Awakening the Sleeping Giant,* as Azmitia titled his review of the subject (Azmitia and Whitaker-Azmitia, 1991), are considerable, given that serotonin has been implicated in a variety of serious clinical conditions, including mood dysregulation, obsessive-compulsive behaviors, eating disorders, sudden infant death syndrome, schizophrenia and Alzheimer's dementia. It might also be worth asking whether the proposed concept of serotonin neuroplasticity could in fact be the basis for an entirely new approach to treating these often unresponsive and refractory conditions. That is, could the loss of certain aspects of serotonergic function actually be at the heart of the proposed therapeutic actions of MDMA? We know, for example, that serotonin neurons in the hippocampus exhibit a high degree of death and regrowth in response to corticosteroid levels. Furthermore, non-neurotoxic decreases in serotonin cause neuroplasticity in adult rats, decreasing the number of nonaminergic synapses in some brain areas (Azmitia, 1999). Within the field of MDMA neurotoxicity, however, Azmitia's theories appear not to have attracted much interest. Although this state of affairs might reflect the politically incorrect nature of even suggesting such a position, there are also issues of safety that cannot be neglected. Indeed, Azmitia's own studies that growth of cultured serotonin cells were stimulated by low concentrations of MDMA but injured at higher concentrations (Azmitia *et al.,* 1990), highlight the need to approach this issue with great caution. Nevertheless, recent awareness of the complexity of these serotonergic systems should spur further discussion of the implications and significance of the changes associated with the phenomenon of MDMA neurotoxicity.

From early on in the debate over MDMA neurotoxicity, the difficulty in demonstrating significant behavioral disturbances in laboratory animals administered large quantities of the drug has remained problematic. In many degenerative brain conditions it is known that 80–90% of the neuronal pathway must be lost for symptoms to appear, as is the case with dopaminergic deficits in Parkinsons Disease. There is no study, however, that has been able to provoke serotonergic losses of that magnitude in response to MDMA treatment, though of course it is not necessarily certain that 5-HT system loss to this degree is necessary for deterioration of clinical function to occur. Even so, there has been the expectation that states of serotonin dysregulation would manifest in disorders of mood, aggression, sexuality, eating, learning and memory. For many years, however, there were virtually no reports of abnormal animal behaviors induced by MDMA. Even those subtle indices of behavioral change which have been identified, however, have not necessarily been evidence of injury. Investigators have reported findings ranging from enhanced conditioned and non-conditioned learning in some animals treated with MDMA (Romano and Harvey, 1993) to attenuation of alcohol consumption in others (Rezvani *et al.*, 1992). Although additional studies have found both slight impairment or no difference compared to control animal function (Slikker *et al.*, 1989; Robinson *et al.*, 1993), the lack of clear proof of injurious functional effect continues to confound the expectations of behavioral consequences in response to neuronal injury by MDMA.

A further cause for concern has been the lack of reports emerging of the long-term effects of high dose MDMA on non-human primate behavior. Recently, Ricaurte and his colleagues reported data describing the immunohistochemical effects in monkeys treated with MDMA seven years previous (Hatzidimitriou *et al.*, 1999). Although that report detailed persistent effects upon neurochemical markers of serotonin function, curiously, there was no discussion of whether behavioral changes occurred. Given the extended period of time Ricuarte and his colleagues maintained the monkeys following their initial treatment with MDMA, seven years previously, one might expect the investigators would have had ample opportunity to observe these non-human primates prior to their eventual destruction, particularly if changes were seen. The field of evolutionary biology is rich with examples of how primate research models have furthered our understanding of the relationship between altered neurotransmitter function and animal behavior, including disorders of mood and aggression (Heinz *et al.*, 1998; Suomi, 1999). The lack of any information on the behavior of these monkeys housed by the investigators for seven years therefore remains puzzling.

Advances have occurred in the field of MDMA neurotoxicity research, leading to clearer understanding of the underlying mechanisms by which high, repeated dosages of MDMA induce serotonergic axonal loss. Several lines of evidence from these investigations suggest a critical role for oxidative stress and the generation of free-radicals that cause degeneration of serotonin axonal terminals (Sprague *et al.,* 1998). It has also been suggested by some investigators that metabolites of MDMA may be involved in the process. Furthermore, multiple neurotransmitter systems appear to exert an influence, as a variety of substances have been demonstrated in laboratory models to be capable of blocking neurotoxicity, including the serotonin reuptake blockers fluoxetine and citalopram (Schmidt, 1987; Schmidt and Taylor, 1987), the serotonin antagonist ritanserin (Schmidt *et al.,* 1990), the dopamine antagonist haloperidol (Hewitt and Green, 1994), the N-methyl-D-aspartate antagonist dizocipline (Colado *et al.,* 1993) and the monoamine oxidase-B inhibitor L-deprenyl (Sprague and Nichols, 1995).

One of the most significant recent achievements investigators in the field have had, however, has been demonstrating the critical role thermoregulatory mechanisms exert on the development of MDMA neurotoxicity. Lewis Seiden, veteran neurotoxicity researcher at the University of Chicago School of Medicine, has reported that relatively small changes in ambient temperature provoke significant alterations in core temperature of MDMA treated rats but do not affect core temperature of control saline treated rats (Malberg and Seiden, 1998). As MDMA neurotoxicity is evidently dependent upon high core temperatures, preventing the development of hyperthermic states in experimental animals will reliably block the loss of serotoninergic terminals (Collado *et al.,* 1995; Broening *et al.,* 1995). The implications of this link between MDMA induced hyperthermia and potential serotonin neurotoxicity to human users are considerable, as temperature is a variable that can be easily regulated. The MDMA treatment paradigm, therefore, appears to be compatible with the imperative to avoid the generation of elevated body temperatures through the use of cool ambient environments, appropriate fluid replacement and the avoidance of physical exertion. On the other hand, the common recreational context of *Ecstasy* use at *raves,* where participants vigorously exer-

cise (dance) for prolonged periods of time often in hot and poorly venti-
lated indoor environments, would appear to heighten risks for MDMA-
induced hyperthermia and magnification of any neurotoxic effect, as well
as for malignant hyperthermia The critical point remains, however, that
MDMA neurotoxicity may be entirely setting dependent and therefore
completely preventable. When considering both the dangers of MDMA
when used as a *rave* drug versus the importance of appropriate temperature control when establishing safety parameters for sanctioned investigations of treatment applications, the importance of these recent laboratory
discoveries of the role of thermoregulation are of great significance to future research developments.

The field of MDMA neurotoxicity research has also taken on the problem of trying to evaluate directly the effects of the drug on humans. Far
more methodologically challenging than animal research, human studies
have often failed to shed much light on the critical questions of MDMA's
effects on health and safety. Indeed, to a regrettable degree, discrepancies
between how studies were actually conducted and how they were reported
in the literature have further clouded an already murky situation. Early
work centered at the Stanford University School of Medicine, where Ricaurte in the late 1980s began to develop his program of human MDMA
neurotoxicity studies. Attempting to investigate whether MDMA decreased levels of the primary metabolite of serotonin in cerebrospinal fluid
(CSF), 5-hydroxyindole acetic acid (5-HIAA), Ricaurte compared a group
of recruited *Ecstasy* users with a control group of chronic pain patients (Ricaurte *et al.*, 1990). Although understandable given human subjects com-
mittee restrictions on conducting lumbar puncture on normal volunteers
in order to obtain CSF, an apparently unrecognized flaw in the design was
that chronic pain is known to induce increased levels of serotonin function, including raised CSF 5-HIAA (Costa *et al.*, 1984; Ceccherelli *et al.*,
1989), thus placing the legitimacy of the findings of relatively low CSF
5-HIAA in *Ecstasy* users into doubt. Although a later report by Ricaurte's
group has repeated the finding (McCann *et al.*, 1994), an earlier investigation from another group found no difference between a smaller sample of
users and nonusers (Peroutka *et al.*, 1989).

A subsequent study, however, raised far more serious questions. Interested in examining MDMA's possible long-term effects on the L-tryptophan challenge model, an indirect measure of serotonin function, a collaborative study was developed by Ricaurte with investigators from Yale University. Publishing their study in the highly prestigious *Archives of General Psychiatry*, the collaborative team reported that MDMA exposure was associated with a trend towards reduced response to L-tryptophan, although the difference between the users and nonusers was not statistically significant (Price *et al.*, 1989). Subsequent scientific reports have sometimes referred to this report as if this difference was significant. What was neither reported in the original article nor corrected by the investigators in the subsequent scientific literature, however, was the fact that the MDMA subjects used in this study were actually pre-selected from the larger group of original Stanford *Ecstasy* users on the basis of their having tested on the lower end of the CSF 5-HIAA spectrum. Utilizing a model of exploring whether markers of serotonin dysfunction are consistent across different tests may be an interesting question, yet given that this was not the purported intent of the study, serious questions about its significance remain (Grob *et al.*, 1990; Grob *et al.*, 1992; Grob and Poland, 1997). Since publication of the article in 1989, it has continued to be regularly cited as a critical piece of evidence for MDMA neurotoxicity in humans.

A logical area of investigation to extrapolate the findings of animal neurotoxicity research to the human model is the neuropsychological influence of presumed MDMA use. Dating back to the late 1980s investigators have conducted evaluations on the cognitive abilities of *Ecstasy* users. The first serious attempt to answer this question occurred in collaboration with the Yale L-tryptophan challenge study. Although concluding that *Ecstasy* users had signs of impaired cognition (Krystal *et al.*, 1992), as with the L-tryptophan study serious questions must be raised concerning basic research design. In addition to the unreported pre-selection subject bias of *Ecstasy* users in the earlier Stanford study who had tested on the low end of the CSF 5-HIAA spectrum, the Yale neuropsychological assessment methodology is also burdened by additional factors which might have predisposed *Ecstasy* subjects to performing less well than their non-Ecstasy using controls. For example, some of the *Ecstasy* subjects were tested the day after flying from the West Coast to New York and several hours after having been administered intravenous L-tryptophan, the serotonin precursor amino acid known to produce sedation in some subjects. Non-*Ecstasy* using literature controls, on the other hand, tend to live locally and therefore are not subjected to cross-country air flight the day before testing. They are also not likely to receive earlier the day of their memory and concentration testing the sedating amino acid serotonin precursor L-tryptophan. In a pre-publication letter to a funder of the investigation, the study neuropsychologist acknowledged that "by and large, these results are striking for the fact that most subjects evaluated had IQ scores in the above average range or higher. Except for the tests mentioned above (Memory and Tactual Performance Test) very few neuropsychological findings exist in this population. It should be noted that the memory findings for the paragraph are not uncommon in patients especially when anxiety, fatigue, or difficulties in attention or concentration exist in the individual. It is quite possible that the large number of impaired scores on the paragraph measures in this population are related to travel fatigue, being in a new environment, or being stressed in some way following the challenge testing that each subject performed" (R. Doblin, pers. com.). The actual published report, however, failed to adequately take into account these important extenuating circumstances. Even though the reported findings of memory impairment were slight and were not clinically significant, and in spite of the suspect methodology, the Yale study has become a cornerstone for the subsequent development of efforts designed to establish the neurotoxic impact of MDMA in humans. While subsequent studies have reported decreased performance in some memory tasks, these decreases are generally less than one standard deviation below the scores of the controls (a difference which is not considered even borderline impairment by clinical neuropsychologists).

Given the degree of risk young people expose themselves to while engaging in the exuberant activities of the *Ecstasy* culture, ranging from polydrug abuse to sleep and nutritional deprivation, there does exist a compelling need to construct and implement psychiatric investigations that will evaluate for signs of injury. Some researchers, particularly neuropsychologists in the United Kingdom, have contributed to our understanding of the short- and long-term effects of marathon drug facilitated dancing on cognition and mood. Valerie Curran, a psychological investigator at the University of London, has described the persistent dysphoria and mild memory impairment experienced by *ravers* during the week following their weekend of drug fueled dancing (Curran and Travill, 1997). These "mid-week lows" were significantly more severe for *Ecstasy* users who were also regular users of cocaine and methamphetamamine. Curran's work, and that of her counterparts in the United Kingdom, have highlighted the degree to which the *Ecstasy* scene has been pervaded with polydrug abuse. In Curran's study, less than two percent of her *Ecstasy* subjects were not polydrug users. An added factor, has been the surge in popularity of the dissociative anesthetic ketamine (Dalgarno and Shewan, 1996). Known to induce strong frontal lobe effects and cognitive dysfunction (Ellison, 1995), ketamine use has increased significantly among *Ecstasy*-using *ravers*. British investigators, to a far greater extent than some of their American counterparts, have been revealing the actual context of *Ecstasy* use experienced by their research subjects. Excessive use of a variety of powerful psychoactive substances, taken at all-night *raves* under conditions of nutritional and sleep deprivation, were all common histories for the *Ecstasy* users recruited into the British studies (Curran, 1998). Although clearly identifing dangers to vulnerable *Ecstasy* culture youth, the investigators acknowledge that these findings tell us far less about the true neuropsychological effects of MDMA.

In the United States, two major studies concluding that MDMA induced memory impairment were published by Ricaurte's group in the late 1990s (Bolla *et al.,* 1998; McCann *et al.,* 1999). Funded by federal grants, the findings of these investigations have received considerable publicity as part of the campaign informing the public that MDMA causes brain damage in humans. Unfortunately, fundamental flaws of research methodology, both reported and unreported, have again obstructed full understanding of what actually occurred. A recurrent problem in Ricaurte's program of retrospective human MDMA research has been his difficulty in providing adequately matched controls. Data published in one study clearly show the far greater exposure of *Ecstasy* subjects to a variety of different drugs when compared to non-*Ecstasy*-using controls, including five times the exposure rates to cocaine and methamphetamine, four times the exposure to PCP and twice the exposure to inhalants. What the report does not provide, however, is the extent to which these different drugs were used by subjects and controls. Given the greater probability that the subjects who had considerable histories of *Ecstasy* ingestion were also far more likely to consume greater quantities of other drugs as well, this discrepancy between the two different groups may well be far more substantial than the published data would indicate. By contrast with the hard-living polydrug-using *Ecstasy* subjects, many controls in these two studies were graduate student volunteers from the local Baltimore-Washington area, a group likely to have had far less exposure to drugs and the *rave* scene. Indeed, "*Ecstasy* use" may be turning into a catchword for a collection of variables that includes the infusion of many drugs into a stressful lifestyle, rather than a characteristic defined by *Ecstasy* use per se.

Other puzzling statistical manipulations have been observed in the study by Bolla *et al* (1998). Although the investigators report that there were no significant differences on memory testing between the 24 *Ecstasy* users and the 24 controls, they nevertheless concluded that "the extent of memory impairment correlates with degree of MDMA exposure." To reach such a conclusion, however, the investigators appear to have used a data chart that was surprisingly excluded from the published report (Nelson, 1999). This ancillary data revealed that in order to demonstrate memory impairment, the subjects had to be divided into a "Control Group," which included not only all 24 controls *but also the 13 subjects with less cumulative Ecstasy use histories,* versus a "High Dose Group," which comprised the remaining 11 subjects with the greater lifetime use of *Ecstasy.* What has been so troubling about this report, published in the peer-reviewed journal *Neurology,* was that neither the number of *Ecstasy* subjects in the high and low dose groups, nor the inclusion of the 13 low-dose *Ecstasy* subjects into a larger control group, were mentioned in the paper. Without these vital data, it is impossible to ascertain how the published findings could have been statistically determined. Even with this knowledge, however, and in spite of well-publicized assertions to the contrary, the evidence from these studies for MDMA-induced memory impairment remains highly suspect.

In late 1998, another study was published purportedly attesting to MDMA's severe dangerousness to humans. Triggering media excitement and concern around the world, the Ricaurte group announced that by means of state-of-the-art Positron Emission Tomography (PET) scans they had identified evidence of "neural injury" in the brains of *Ecstasy* users (McCann *et al.*, 1998). Uncritically accepting his conclusions as reported in the highly regarded British journal *Lancet,* the world press followed the lead of the *Times of London,* which announced on October 30, 1998, that Ricaurte had definitively demonstrated "Proof That *Ecstasy* Damages The Brain." Under close scrutiny, however, both the methodology and data interpretation employed by this particular study appear to suffer from some of the same limitations exposed in his earlier work. Although the rapidly progressing field of modern brain-imaging techniques offers great potential to aid our understanding of MDMA's effects on the brain, including the concern over possible neural damage, this most recent contribution from the Ricaurte team once again raises more questions than it answers.

Utilizing a recently developed technique to visualize components of the serotonin neurotransmitter system, Ricaurte attempted to demonstrate abnormal findings in a group of 14 *Ecstasy*-using subjects compared with a second group of 15 normal controls who had never used *Ecstasy.* Essential data characterizing these two groups, however, is missing. Although the investigators say they administered a drug-history questionnaire to their subjects, these critical results are absent from the report. No information is therefore provided addressing the critical question of polydrug abuse among *Ecstasy* users. The degree to which these subjects may have had exposure to methamphetamine, cocaine, opiates, barbiturates, hallucinogens, ketamine, PCP, cannabis, inhalants, tobacco, alcohol or other substances in addition to *Ecstasy*, does not enter into the authors' interpretation of their reported data (Erowid, 1998a). Nor is there any discussion of the poly-morphous nature of *Ecstasy* itself, that in addition to being MDMA it might also constitute other drugs, including MDA, MDE, MBDB, 2CB, methamphetamine, LSD, psilocybin, ketamine, PCP or dextromethor-phan. Simply put by Ricaurte, the study succeeds in demonstrating the in-jurious effects of MDMA on the brain serotonin system. On closer inspection of the research design employed, however, it is apparent that by choosing subjects who reported taking *Ecstasy* on an average of 228 (70–400) separate occasions, 6 (1–16) times per month for 4.6 (1.5–10.0) years, the investigators were selecting a group of unarguably heavy users of *Ecstasy*. Indeed, the average dose of presumed MDMA reportedly taken by the subjects, 386 (150–1250) milligrams, is an exceptionally large amount, approximately three times the recommended therapeutic dose. It is diffi-cult to believe that *Ecstasy* was the only drug used in high doses by these subjects. Given these inherent problems in methodological controls, at-tempts to extrapolate to the occasional (or one-time) low dose MDMA treatment model remain highly problematic.

For the PET technique used by the Ricaurte group, each subject was in-jected with a radioactive labeled marker that selectively binds to serotonin (5-HT) transporters (the serotonin re-uptake sites) on the axons of sero-tonin neurons. These transporters consist of protein structures that are embedded in the membranes of nerve endings and are part of the in-terneuron communication system. The key finding, reported in the study, was that MDMA users showed decreased global and regional brain sero-tonin transporter-binding compared with controls. Reporting that de-creases in serotonin transporter-binding positively correlated with the extent of previous *Ecstasy* use, the authors conclude by stating that they had demonstrated "direct evidence of a decrease in a structural compo-nent of brain 5-HT neurons in human MDMA users." Closer examination of the research design and method of data interpretation employed, how-ever, reveals serious shortcomings. First, the identified MDMA users hardly appear to have abnormally low-serotonin transporter levels at all. Looking at the data chart provided, it is clear that there is relatively little difference between the subject group and the control group. Only one of the *Ecstasy* users falls well outside the range of the rest of the subjects. Excluding that particular individual (with a reported life-time total of 150 *Ecstasy* ingestions), all of the remaining presumed MDMA users' scores are within the same range as the non-MDMA users. As 2 of the 14 MDMA users are actually near the top of the non-MDMA user range (and above the majority of controls), confidence that these data support the findings remains lacking. Indeed, if one removes the one outlier subject and the 15 controls who had been included to weight the correlation curve, a new regression analysis reveals no statistically significant correlation between MDMA use and transporter density. The touted effect correlating low transporter and MDMA use appears to disappear altogether (Erowid, 1998b). Finally, disregard of the possibility that some subjects may have had pre-existing low transporter levels prior to initial *Ecstasy* exposure, perhaps even predisposing them to polydrug abuse to begin with, further erodes the significance of the reported findings.

Doubts have also been raised about the experimental PET approach used in the study, the [11C]–McNeil-5652 serotonin ligand, which has only recently been available to investigators. Only a handful of brain imaging researchers have had access to this developing technology, including two groups of European investigators who have commented critically on the technique used by the Ricaurte group. Professors Kuikka and Ahonen at the Universities of Kuopio and Oulu in Finland have responded to the original article in *Lancet* that the approach used in that study raises the question of whether the reported reductions in serotonin transporter are in fact actually based on different kinetics of the non-specific radioligand [11C]–McNeil-5652 between controls and presumed MDMA users (Kuikka and Ahonen, 1999). The other group that has raised questions about Ricaurte's PET methodology, at the University of Zurich under the leadership of Franz Vollenweider, has been at the forefront of the recent resurgence of high-level European neuropsychiatric research with hallucinogens and phenethylamines, including MDMA. Having considerable experience with brain imaging and the [11C)–McNeil-5652 ligand, Vollenweider has emphasized that test-retest variability must first be assessed in order to know how stable and reliable the data actually are (Buck *et al.,* 2000; F.X. Vollenweider, pers. com.). The failure of Ricaurte and his colleagues to account for and report the test-retest variability for their technique further underscores the degree to which methodological uncertainty persists with the particular PET scanning approach used.

Finally, there remains the question of what a reduction of serotonin transporters means, if MDMA is capable of inducing such an effect. Does a decrease in measurable transporter density inevitably mean structural damage to the serotonin system? Or, might it simply be a reflection of a functional modulation (pharmacologic downregulation) in response to lower concentrations of the neurotransmitter. Neuronal systems are known to be capable of exhibiting a wide range of adaptive and compensatory responses in response to toxic effects or drug use. In recent years, the classical view of antidepressant drugs as modulators of acute synaptic events has been broadened to include long-term actions that modify neuronal function. Administration of serotonin ligands, including tricyclic and selective reuptake-inhibiting antidepressants, have been shown to reduce significantly both the expression of serotonin transporter mRNA as well as the density of serotonin transporter-binding sites labeled by [3H]paroxetine in the dorsal raphe nuceus in rats (Lesch *et al.,* 1993; Watanabe *et al.,* 1993; Kuroda *et al.,* 1994). Interestingly, the recreational drug cocaine has also been shown to decrease significantly the abundance of serotonin transporter mRNA (Burchett and Bannon, 1997). To buttress their contention that MDMA is a dangerous human neurotoxin, Ricaurte and his colleagues have charged that the failure to observe severe short-term negative clinical sequelae is deceptive, and that it might take years for neuropsychiatric signs of serotonin to manifest (the "Time Bomb" theory of MDMA neurotoxicity). They introduce the example of the dopamine neurotoxin MPTP into the argument, and describe how with age the functional dopamine reserve must be progressively depleted before individuals become symptomatic with Parkinson's Disease. What they fail to acknowledge, however, is that unlike the dopamine system, which clearly declines with advancing age in humans and animals, the serotonin neurotransmitter system appears to maintain relative stability over time with significantly lesser degrees of chronological decline than the case of dopamine (McEntee and Cook, 1991). Although legitimate concerns remain that heavy *Ecstasy* users may have caused long-standing alterations in their central nervous system function by their life style and drug-taking habits, the Ricaurte PET data sheds little light on the range of MDMA's effects on humans.

Current Status

During the concluding years of the twentieth century and into the twenty-first century, *Ecstasy* use has continued to spread throughout the United States and Europe. Increasing numbers of youth, at younger ages, are attending *raves* where the vast majority ingest a variety of drugs. The reliability of *Ecstasy* supplies has continued to deteriorate, highlighting the poor quality control which exists on the illicit drug market. The trend for drugs other than MDMA to be used as substitutes for *Ecstasy* has intensified, typified by a recent report from the French *rave* scene identifying that only 25% of *Ecstasy* pills analyzed by *Medicins du Monde* representatives actually contained MDMA (Inciyan, 2000). A variety of different drugs, often but not necessarily disguised as *Ecstasy,* are now in wide circulation on the youth recreational drug market, including methamphetamine, cocaine, opiates, hallucinogens, inhalants, PCP, ketamine, dextramethorphan and GHB. To fully appreciate the degree of public health risk, it is essential for investigators to acknowledge the polydrug context of *Ecstasy* culture. To mistake the cumulative consequences of multiple drug use for the effects of MDMA alone obfuscates our understanding of this complex phenomenon.

The implications to millions of youth world-wide frequently self-administering these powerful psychoactive drugs remain unclear. Virtually all research efforts to date have been directed at establishing through laboratory animal investigations and retrospective human *Ecstasy* user models the neurotoxic dangers of MDMA. After 15 years, however, the case has yet to be made. Although long-term alterations of neuronal architecture in animals ranging from rats to non-human primates have been consistently demonstrated, the functional consequences have remained obscure. Furthermore, efforts to extrapolate evidence of MDMA-induced neuropathology from retrospective examinations of heavy *Ecstasy* users have consistently manifested serious methodologic flaws. Although laboratory experimentation in particular has provided fertile ground for the advancement of our knowledge of brain neurotransmitter systems, the MDMA neurotoxicity research model, media hype aside, has demonstrated limited clinical utility.

While the dangers youth expose themselves to while engaged in the activities of *Ecstasy* culture should by no means be written off lightly, more objective appraisal of risk for the long neglected low-dose MDMA treatment model needs to be examined. Relying on evaluation of youth with extensive polydrug histories, extreme lifestyles and often comorbid psychopatholgies to inform us of the effects of MDMA imposes an inadequate and misleading perspective. The only way to rigorously establish true risk (and safety) parameters is to utilize prospective human research models. Only by administering known quantities of pure drug in a research setting controlling for extraneous factors (including though not limited to ancillary drug use), will we be able to establish an accurate profile of MDMA's effects. In spite of the compelling need to utilize human administration research models, however, only a handful of studies have been conducted. For years, fears aroused by the publicization of neurotoxicity concerns have stalled the development of alternative research paradigms. Although a limited number of prospective investigations have been permitted, recent efforts to expand such research programs (Vollenweider *et al.*, 1998; Vollenweider *et al.*, 1999; Lieberman and Aghajanian, 1999) have come under dubious attack (Gijsman *et al.*, 1999; McCann and Ricaurte, 2000). While clearly strong human subject protection procedures must be assured for all investigations of this sort, a process of truly objective risk assessment should allow for the cautious elaboration of these optimal research models.

With the brief and isolated exception of the Swiss psycholytic group experience ten years ago, there has been no authorized treatment since MDMA was classified as a Schedule I drug in the mid-1980s. The regulatory decision to allow a formal program to investigate the safety and efficacy of MDMA as a treatment modality has not as yet been reached, although there have been hopeful signs for the future. Indeed, a growing consensus is beginning to recognize the need to conduct prospective research with pharmaceutical-grade MDMA on subjects who are neither denizens of *Ecstasy* culture nor severe polysubstance abusers. There is no doubt that recreational *Ecstasy* users are exposing themselves to greater and more unusual risks than were ever anticipated by the early explorers of MDMA's putative therapeutic effects (Jansen, 1998, Brody *et al.,* 1998; Harrington *et al.,* 1999). And yet, what is the genuine relevance to the clinical treatment model of such poorly controlled data collected from populations of young polydrug users who have frequented for extended periods of time the fast lane of the contemporary *rave* scene? Hopefully, the time has arrived where it will be possible to undertake sanctioned studies which will finally and honestly elucidate the true risk/benefit ratio for this misunderstood drug.

The world of contemporary *Ecstasy* use poses many dangers for our youth. Exposed to the vagaries of the underground drug trade, and misguided by the omnipotence and naivete of their age, millions of young people experimenting with today's panoply of substances have ignored their elders' admonitions of caution and have continued to pursue the activities of *Ecstasy* culture. Denied the safeguards provided to youth initiates of traditional cultures, young *ravers* in our own contemporary world continue to incur unnecessary degrees of risk (Grob and DeRios, 1992; DeRios and Grob, 1994). Clearly, new models for assessing the unique properties of MDMA, both positive and negative, are called for. The old models which have stalled the development of alternative paradigms, have also unfortunately impeded the flow of open and honest dialogue on these critical issues. The long-neglected treatment model of MDMA-augmented psychotherapy has to date neither been disproven nor proven. Particularly in patients with severe refractory conditions, including the psychological distress associated with end-stage cancer and the spectrum of chronic post-traumatic stress disorder, rigorous and well-controlled research assessment of safety and efficacy deserves investigation. Utilizing thorough and comprehensive informed consent procedures, strict standards of medical ethics should be satisfied. Hopefully, the opportunity now exists to develop and implement those research models which will finally address not only the pressing public health concerns implicit within modern *Ecstasy* culture, but also the never-answered questions of MDMA's potential as a therapeutic medicine.

References

Adamson, S. (1985). *Through the Gateway of the Heart: Accounts of Experiences with MDMA and Other Empathogenic Substances.* San Francisco: Four Trees Publications.

Adamson, S. and Metzner, R. (1988). The nature of the MDMA experience and its role in healing, psychotherapy and spiritual practice. *ReVision,* **10,** 59–72.

Ali, S. F., Newport, G. D., Scallet, A. C., Binienda, Z., Ferguson, S. A. and Bailey, J. R. (1993). Oral administration of MDMA produces selective 5-HT depletion in the non-human primate. *Neurotoxicol Teratol.,* **15,** 91–96.

Azmitia, E. C., Murphy, R. B. and Whitaker-Azmitia, P. M. (1990). MDMA (Ecstasy) effects on cultured serotonergic neurons: evidence for Ca^{++} dependent toxicity linked to release. *Brain Res.,* **510,** 97–103.

Azmitia, E. C. and Whitaker-Azmitia, P. M. (1991). Awakening the sleeping giant: anatomy and plasticity of the brain serotonergic system. *J. Clin. Psychiatry,* **52** (suppl), 4–16.

Bakalar, J. and Grinspoon, J. B. (1990). *Testing psychotherapies and drug therapies: the case of psychedelic drugs.* In: S. J. Peroutka, (Ed.). Ecstasy: The Clinical, Pharmacological and Neurotoxicological Effects of the Drug MDMA. Holland: Kluwer, pp. 37–52.

Battaglia, G., Yeh, S. Y. and DeSouza, E. B. (1988). MDMA-induced neurotoxicity: parameters of degeneration and recovery of brain serotonin neurons. *Pharmacol. Biochem. Behav.,* **29,** 269–274.

Beck, J. (1993). Ecstasy and the rave scene: historical and cross-cultural perspectives. *CEWG* Dec: 424–431.

Beck, J. and Morgan, P. A. (1986). Designer drug confusion: a focus on MDMA. *J. Drug Education.* **16,** 287–302.

Beck, J. and Rosenbaum, M. (1994) *Pursuit of Ecstasy: The MDMA Experience.* State University of New York Press: Albany, New York.

Bolla, K. I., McCann, U. D. and Ricaurte, G. A. (1998). Memory impairment in abstinent MDMA ("Ecstasy") users. *Neurology.* **51,** 1532–1537.

Brody, S., Krause, Veit, R. and Rau, H. (1998). Cardiovascular autonomic dysregulation users of MDMA ("ecstasy"). *Psychopharmacol.,* **136,** 390–393.

Broening, H. W., Bowyer, J. F. and Slikker, W. (1995). Age-dependent sensitivity of rats to the long-term effects of the serotonergic neurotoxicant (±)3,4-methylenedioxymethampethamine (MDMA) correlates with the magnitude of the MDMA-induced thermal response. *J. Pharmacol. Exp. Ther.,* **275,** 325–333.

Buchanan, J. F. and Brown, C. R. (1988). Designer drugs: a problem in clinical toxicology. *Med. Toxicol.,* **3,** 1–17.

Buck, A., Gucker, P., Vollenweider, F. X. and Burger, C. (2000). Evaluation of serotonergic transporter using PET and 11C-(+)-McN-5652: assessment of methods. *J. Cerebral Blood Flow Metabolism,* in press.

Burchett, S. A. and Bannon, M. J. (1997). Serotonin, dopamine and norepinephrine transporter mRNAs: heterogeneity of distribution and response to 'binge' cocaine administration. *Molecular Brain Res.,* **49,** 95–102.

Burger, A. J., Sherman, H. B., Charlamb, M. J., Kim, J., Asinas, L. A., Flickner, S. R. and Blackburn, G. L. (1999). Low prevalence of valvular heart disease in 226 phenterminefenfluramine protocol subjects prospectively followed for up to 30 months. *J. Am. Coll. Cardiol.,* **34,** 1153–1158.

Caccia, S., Ballabio, M., Guiso, G., Rochetti, M. and Garattini, S. (1982). Species differences in the kinetics of metabolism of fenfluramine isomers. *Arch. Int. Pharmacodyn.,* **258,** 15–28.

Caccia, S., Anelli, M., Ferrarese, A., Fracasso, C. and Garattini, S. (1993). The role of d-norfenfluramine in the indole-depleting effect of d-fenfluramine in the rat. *Eur. J. Pharmacol.,* **223,** 71–77.

Capdevila, M. (1995). *MDMA o el Extasis Quimico.* Barcelona: Los Libros De La Liebre De Marzo.

Ceccherelli, F., Costa, C., Ischia, S., Ischia, A., Giron, G. and Alletri, G. (1989). Cerebral tryptophan metabolism in humans in relation to malignant pain. *Funct. Neurol.,* **4,** 341–353.

Chappell, S. and Mordenti, J. (1991). *Extrapolation of toxicological and pharmacological data from animals to humans.* In B. Tests, (Ed.). Advances in Drug Research. San Diego: Academic Press, pp. 1–116.

Colado, M. I., Murray, T. K. and Green, A. R. (1993). 5-HT loss in rat brain following 3,4-methylenedioxymethamphetamine (MDMA), p-chloroamphetamine and fenfluramine administration and effects of chlormethiazole and dizocilpine. *Br. J. Pharmacol.,* **108,** 583–589.

Colado, M. I., Williams, J. L. and Green, A. R. (1995). The hyperthermic and neurotoxic effects of "Ecstasy" (MDMA) and 3,4-methylenedioxyamphetamine (MDA) in the Dark Agouti (DA) rat, a model of the CYP2D6 poor metabolizer phenotype. *Br. J. Pharmacol.,* **115,** 1281–1289.

Collin, M. (1998). *Altered State: The Story of Ecstasy Culture and Acid House.* London: Serpent's Tail.

Costa, C., Ceccherelli, F., Bettero, A., Marin, G., Mancusi, L. and Allegri, G. (1984). *Tryptophan, serotonin and 5-hydroxyindoleacetic acid levels in human CSF in relation to pain.* In H. G. Schlossberger, W. Kochen, B. Linzen and H. Steinhart, (Eds.). Progress in Tryptophan and Serotonin Research, pp. 413–416

Cuomo, J. J., Dyment, P. G. and Gammino, V. M. (1994). Increasing use of "ecstasy" (MDMA) and other hallucinogens of a college campus. *J. Amer. College Health Assoc.,* **42,** 271–274.

Curran, H. V. (1998). *Is ecstasy (MDMA) a human neurotoxin?* Novartis Foundation Conference. London, December 4.

Curran, H. V. and Travill, R. A. (1997). Mood and cognitive effects of ±3,4-methylenedioxymethamphetamine (MDMA, 'ecstasy'): week-end 'high' followed by mid-week low. *Addiction.* **92,** 821–831.

Dalgarno, P .J. and Shewan, D. (1996). Illicit use of ketamine in Scotland. *J. Psychoactive Drugs,* **28,** 191–199.

DeRios, M. D. and Grob, C. S. (1994). Hallucinogens, suggestibility and adolescence in cross-cultural perspective. *Yearbook Ethnomedicine,* **3,** 113–132.

Derome-Tremblay, M. and Nathan, C. (1989). Fenfluramine studies. *Science.* **243,** 991.

Doblin, R. (1996). MAPS MDMA analysis project. *MAPS,* **6,** 11–13.

Dowling, G. P., McDonough, E. T. and Bost, R. O. (1987). "Eve" and "ecstasy": a report of five deaths associated with the use of MDEA and MDMA. *JAMA,* **257,** 1615–1617.

Downing, J. (1986). The psychological and physiological effects of MDMA on normal volunteers. *J. Psychoactive Drugs,* **18,** 335–339.

Eisner, B. (1989). *Ecstasy: The MDMA Story.* Berkeley: Ronin Publishing.

Eliade, M. (1951). *Shamanism: Archaic Techniques of Ecstasy.* Paris: Librarie Payot.

Ellison, G. (1995). The N-methyl-D-aspartate antagonists phencyclidine, ketamine and dizocilpine as both behavioral and anatomical models of dementias. *Brain Res. Rev.,* **20,** 250–267.

Erowid, E. (1998a). *Comments on MDMA neurotoxicity study: a prospective guinea pig.* http://www.erowid.org?chemicals/mdma/mdma_journal3/mdma_journal3_comment3.shtml.

Erowid E. (1998b). *MDMA neurtoxicity study: questioning the correlation between increased MDMA use and decreased binding—an analysis of figure 4 of the McCann-Ricaurte MDMA study results.* http://www.erowid.org/chemicals/mdma/mdma_journal3_statistics.shtml.

Furnari, C., Ottaviano, V., Rosati, F. and Tondi, V. (1998). Identification of 3,4-methylenedioxymethamphetamine analogs encountered in clandestine tablets. *Forensic Science International,* **92,** 49–58.

Gasser, P. (1995a). Die psycholytische psychotherapie in der Schweiz (1988–1993). *Jahrbuch fur Transkulturelle Medizin und Psychotherapie,* **6,** 143–162.

Gasser, P. (1995b). The psycholytic therapy in Switzerland from 1988–1993: a follow-up study. *MAPS,* **5,** 3–7.

Gijsman, G., Vrekes, R., van Gervan, J. and Cohen, A. (1999). MDMA study. *Neuropsychopharmacol.,* **21,** 597.

Greer, G. and Tolbert, R. (1986). Subjective reports of the effects of MDMA in a clinical setting. *J. Psychoactive Drugs,* **18,** 319–327.

Grinspoon, L. and Bakalar, J. B. (1979). *Psychedelic Drugs Reconsidered.* New York: Basic Books.

Grinspoon, L. and Bakalar, J. B. (1986). Can drugs be used to enhance the psychotherapeutic process? *Am. J. Psychotherapy,* **40,** 393–404.

Grob, C. S. (1998). Psychiatric research with hallucinogens: what have we learned? *Heffter. Rev. Psychedelic Research,* **1,** 8–20.

Grob, C. S. and DeRios, M. D. (1992). Adolescent drug use in cross-cultural perspective. *J. Drug Issues,* **22,** 121–138.

Grob, C. S. and Poland, R. E. (1997). MDMA. In J. H. Lowinson, P. Ruiz, R. B. Millman, and J. G. Langrod, (Eds). *Substance Abuse: A Comprehensive Textbook,* Third Edition. Baltimore: Williams and Wilkins, pp. 269–275.

Grob, C. S., Bravo, G. L. and Walsh, R. N. (1990). Second thoughts on 3,4-methylenedioxymethamphetamine (MDMA) neurotoxicity. *Arch. Gen. Psychiatry,* **47,** 288.

Grob, C. S., Bravo, G. L., Walsh, R. N. and Liester, M. B. (1992). The MDMA-neurotoxicity controversy: implications for clinical research with novel psychoactive drugs. *J. Nerv. Ment. Dis.,* **180,** 355–356.

Grob, C. S., Poland, R. E., Chang, L. and Ernst, T. (1996). Psychobiologic effects of 3,4-methylenedioxymethamphetamine in humans: methodological considerations and preliminary findings. *Behav. Brain Research,* **73,** 103–107.

Harrington, R. D., Woodward, J. A., Hooton, T. M. and Horn, J. R. (1999). Life-threatening interactions between HIV-1 protease inhibitors and the illicit drugs MDMA and gamma-hydroxybutyrate. *Arch. Intern. Med.,* **159,** 2221–2224.

Harris Research Center (1992). Young people's poll.

Harris, D., Baggott, Jones, R. T. and Mendelson, J. (1999). MDMA pharmacokinetics and physiological and subjective effects in humans. *CPDD,* 59.

Harvey, J. A., McMaster, S. E. and Yunger, L. M. (1975). p-Chloroamphetamine: selective neurotoxic action in brain. *Science,* **187,** 841–843.

Hatzidimitriou, G., McCann, U. D. and Ricaurte, G. A. (1999). Altered serotonin innervation patterns in the forebrain of monkeys treated with MDMA seven years previously: factors influencing abnormal recovery. *J. Neurosci.,* **191,** 5096–5107.

Heinz, A., Higley, J. D., Gorey, J. G., Saunders, R. C., Jones, D. W., Hommer, D., Zajicek, K., Suomi, S. J., Lesch, K. P., Weinberger, D. R. and Linnoila, M. (1998). In vivo association between alcohol intoxication, aggression, and serotonin transporter availability in nonhuman primates. *Am. J. Psychiatry,* **155,** 1023–1028.

Henry, J. A., Jeffreys, K. J. and Dawling, S. (1992). Toxicity and deaths from 3,4-methlyenedioxymethamphetamine ("ecstasy"). *Lancet,* **340,** 384–387.

Hekmatpanah, C. R. and Peroutka, S. J. (1990). 5-hydroxytryptamine uptake blockers attenuate the 5-hydroxytryptamine-releasing effect of 3,4-methylenedioxymethamphetamine and related agents. *Eur. J. Pharmacol.,* **177,** 95–98.

Hewitt, K. E. and Green, A. R. (1994). Chlormethiazole, dizocilpine and haloperidol prevent the degeneration of serotonergic nerve terminals induced by administration of MDMA ("Ecstasy"). *Neuropharmacol.,* **33,** 1589–1595.

Inciyan, E. (2000). Ecstasy's high-risk agenda. *The Guardian,* February 24.

Jansen, K. L. R. (1998). Ecstasy (MDMA) dependence. *Drug Alcohol Dependence,* **53,** 121–124.

Johnson, M. P. and Nichols, D. E. (1990). Comparative serotonin neurotoxicity of the steroisomers of fenfluramine and norfenfluramine. *Pharmacol. Biochem. Behav.,* **36,** 105–109.

Karel, R. (1993). Fluoxetine may protect against MDMA neurotoxicity. *Psychiatric News,* August 6.

King, L. A. (1998). Comments. Novartis Foundation Conference: *Is Ecstasy (MDMA) A Human Neurotoxin?* London, December 4.

Krystal, J. H., Price, L. H., Opsahl, C., Ricaurte, G. A. and Heninger, G. R. (1992). Chronic 3,4-methylenedioxymethamphetamine (MDMA) use: effects on mood and neuropsychological function? *Am. J. Drug Alcohol Abuse,* **18,** 331–341.

Kuikka, J. T. and Ahonen, A. K. (1999). Letter on toxic effect of MDMA on brain serotonin neurons. *Lancet,* **353,** 1269.

Kuroda, Y., Watanabe, Y. and McEwen, B. S. (1994). Tianeptine decreases both serotonin transporter mRNA and binding sites in rat brain. *Eur. J. Pharmacol.,* **268,** R3–R5.

Lawn, J. C. (1986). Schedules of controlled substances: scheduling of 3,4-methylenedioxymethamphetamine (MDMA) into Schedule I. *Federal Register,* **51,** 36552–36560.

Lesch, K. P., Aulakh, C. S., Wolozin, B. L., Tolliver, T. J., Hill, J. L. and Murphy, D. L. (1993). Regional brain expression of serotonin transporter mRNA and its regulation by reuptake-inhibiting antidepressants. *Molecular Brain Res.,* **17,** 31–35.

Lieberman, J. and Aghajanian, G. (1999). Caveat emptor: researcher beware. *Neuropsychopharmacol.,* **21,** 472.

Malberg, J. E. and Seiden, L. S. (1998). Small changes in ambient temperature cause large changes in 3,4-methylenedioxymethamphetamine (MDMA)-induced serotonin neurotoxicity and core body temperature in the rat. *J. Neurosci.,* **18,** 5086–5094.

Manchanda, S. and Connolly, M. J. (1993). Cerebral infarction in association with ecstasy abuse. *Postgrad Med. J.,* **69,** 874–879.

Marchant, M. C., Breen, M. A., Wallace, D., Bass, S., Taylor, A. R., Ings, R. M. J. and Campbell, B. (1992). Comparative biodisposition and metabolism of 14C-(+/–)-fenfluramine in mouse, rat, dog and man. *Xenobiotica,* **12,** 1251–1266.

Mas, M., Farre, M., De La Torre, R., Roset, P. N., Ortuno, J., Segura, J. and Cami, J. (1999). Cardiovascular and neuroendocrine effects and pharmacokinetics of 3,4-methylenedioxymethamphetamine in humans. *J. Pharmacol. Exp. Ther.,* **290,** 136–145.

Matthews, A. and Jones, C. (1992). Spate of British ecstasy deaths puzzles experts. *Int. J. Drug Policy,* **3,** 4.

McCann, U. D. and Ricaurte, G. A. (1995). On the neurotoxicity of MDMA and related amphetamine derivatives. *J. Clin. Psychopharmacol.,* **15,** 295–296.

McCann, U. D. and Ricaurte, G. A. (2000). Caveat emptor: editors beware. *Neuropsychopharmacology,* in press.

McCann, U., Hatzidimitriou, G., Ridenour, A., Fischer, C., Yuan, J., Katz, J. and Ricaurte, G. (1994). Dexfenfluramine and serotonin neurotoxicity: further preclinical evidence that clinical caution is indicated. *J. Pharmacol. Exp. Ther.,* **269,** 792–798.

McCann, U. D., Mertl, M., Eligulashvili, V. and Ricaurte, G. A. (1999). Cognitive performance in (±)3,4-methylenedioxymethamphetamine (MDMA, "ecstasy") users: a controlled study. *Psychpharmacol.,* **143,** 417–425.

McCann, U. D., Szabo, Z., Scheffel, U., Dannals, R. F. and Ricaurte, G. A. (1998). Positron emission tomographic evidence of toxic effect of MDMA ("ecstasy") on brain serotonin neurons in human beings. *Lancet,* **352,** 1433–1437.

McEntee, W. J. and Crook, T. H. (1991). Serotonin, memory and the aging brain. *Psychopharmacol.,* **103,** 143–149.

McKenna, D.J. and Peroutka, S.J. (1990). Neurochemistry and neurotoxicity of 3,4-methylenedioxymethamphetamine. *J. Neurochem.,* **54,** 14–22.

Molliver, M. E., Berger, U. V., Mamounas, L. A., Molliver, D. C., O'Hearn, E. and Wilson, M. A. (1990). Neurotoxicity of MDMA and related compounds: anatomic studies. *Ann. NY Acad. Sci.,* **600,** 640–664.

Nelson, K. T. (1999). MDMA and memory impairment: proven or not? *MAPS,* **9**(3), 6–8.

Newmeyer, J. A. (1993). X at the crossroads. *J. Psychoactive Drugs,* **25,** 341–342.

NIDA Capsules (1993). CAP 16, U.S. Department of Health and Human Services, National Institute on Drug Abuse.

NIDA [1999] www.monitoringthefuture.org

O'Callaghan, J. P. (1993). Quantitative features of reactive gliosis following toxicant-induced damage to the CNS. *Ann. N. Acad. Sci.,* **679,** 195–210.

O'Callaghan, J. P. (1995). Commentary on article by Ricaurte and colleagues. *MAPS,* **6**(1), 13.

O'Callaghan, J. P. and Miller, D. B. (1993). Quantification of reactive gliosis as an approach to neurotoxicity assessment. In Erinoff, L. (Ed.). *Assessing Neurotoxicity of Drugs of Abuse*. National Institute on Drug Abuse Monograph 136, Washington, D.C: U.S. Government Printing Office, 188–212.

O'Callaghan, J. P. and Miller, D. B. (1994). Neurotoxicity profiles of substituted amphetamines in the C57BL/6J mouse. *J. Pharmacol. Exp. Ther.,* **270,** 741–751.

Parrott, A. (1998). *Is ecstasy (MDMA) a human neurotoxin?* Novartis Foundation Conference. London, December 4.

Peroutka, S. J. (1987). Incidence of recreational use of 3,4-methlenedioxymethamphetamine (MDMA, "ecstasy") on an undergradulate campus. *New England J. Med.,* **317,** 1542–1543.

Peroutka, S. J. (1988). Relative insensitivity of mice to 3,4-methylenedioxymethamphetamine neurotoxicity. *Res. Commun. Subs. Abuse.,* **9,** 193–206.

Pletscher, A., Burkar, W. P., Bruderer, H. and Gey, K. F. (1963). Decrease of cerebral 5-hydroxytryptamine and 5-hydroxyindolacetic acid by arylalkylamine. *Life Sci.,* **11,** 828–833.

Price, L. H., Ricaurte, G. A., Krystal, J. H. and Henninger, G. R. Neuroendocrine and mood responses to intravenous l-tryptophan in 3,4-methylenedioxymethamphetamine (MDMA) users. *Arch. Gen. Psychiatry,* **46,** 20–22.

Randall, T. (1992). Ecstasy-fuled "rave" parties become dances of death for English youths. *JAMA,* **268,** 1505–1506.

Rezvani, A. H., Garges, P. L., Miller, D. B. and Gordon, C. J. (1992). Attenuation of alcohol consumption by MDMA (Ecstasy) in two strains of alcohol-preferring rats. *Pharmacol. Biochem. Behav.,* **43,** 103–110.

Ricaurte, G., Bryan, G., Strauss, L., Seiden, L. and Schuster, C. (1985). Hallucinogenic amphetamine selectively destroys brain serotonin nerve terminals. *Science,* **229,** 986–988.

Ricaurte, G. A., Finnegan, K. T., Irwin, I. and Langston, J. W. (1990). Aminergic metabolites in cerebrospinal fluid of humans previously exposed to MDMA: preliminary observations. *Ann. NY Acad. Sci.,* **600,** 699–708.

Riedlinger, T. J. and Riedlinger, J. E. (1994). Psychedelic and entactogenic drugs in the treatment of depression. *J. Psychoactive Drugs,* **26,** 41–55.

Robinson, T. E., Castandea, E. and Whishaw, I. Q. (1993). Effects of cortical serotonin depletion induced by 3,4-methylenedioxymethamphetamine (MDMA) on behavior, before and after additional cholinergic blockade. *Neuropsychopharmacol.,* **8,** 77–85.

Romano, A. G. and Harvey, J. A. (1993). MDMA enhances associative and nonassociative learning in the rabbit. *Pharmacol. Biochem. Behav.,* **47,** 289–293.

Sanders-Bush, E., Bushing, J. A. and Sulser, F. (1975). Long-term effects of p-chloroamphetamine and related drugs of central serotonergic mechanisms. *J. Pharmacol. Exp. Ther.,* **192,** 33–40.

Saunders, N. (1993). *E for Ecstasy.* London: Saunders.

Saunders, N. (1995). *Ecstasy and the dance culture.* London: Saunders.

Saunders, N. and Doblin, R. (1996). *Ecstasy: Dance Trance and Transformation.* Oakland, California: Quick American Archives.

Schifano, F., DiFuria, L., Forz, G., Minicuci, N. and Bricolo, R. (1998). MDMA ('ecstasy') consumption in the context of polydrug abuse: a report on 150 patients. *Drug Alcohol Dependence,* **52,** 85–90.

Schiller, N. B. (1999). Fen/phen and valvular heart disease: if it sounds too bad to be true, perhaps it isn't. *J. Am. Coll. Cardiol.,* **34,** 1159–1162.

Schmidt, C. J. (1987). Neurotoxicity of the psychedelic amphetamine, methylenedioxymethamphetamine. *J. Pharmacol. Exp. Ther.,* **240,** 1–7.

Schmidt, C. J. and Taylor, V. L. (1987). Depression of rat brain tryptophan hydroxylase following the acute administration of methylenedioxymethamphetamine. *Biochem. Pharmacol.,* **36,** 4095–4102.

Schmidt, C. J., Abbate, G. M., Black, C. K. and Taylor, V. L. (1990). Selective 5-HT2 receptor antagonists protect against the neurotoxicity of methylenedioxymethamphetamine in rats. *J. Pharmacol. Exp. Ther.,* **255,** 478–483.

Schultes, R. E. and Hofmann, A. (1992). *Plants of the Gods: Their Sacred, Healing and Hallucinogenic Powers.* Rochester, Vermont: Healing Arts Press.

Sferios, E. (1999). Report from DanceSafe: laboratory analysis program reveals DXM tablets sold as "ecstasy." *MAPS Bull,* **9**(4), 47.

Sharkey A. (1996). Sorted or distorted. *The Guardian,* 26 January: 2–4.

Shewan, D., Dalgarno, P. and King, L. A. (1996). Tablets often contain substances in addition to, or instead of, ecstasy. *Lancet,* **313,** 423–424.

Shulgin, A. T. (1986) The background and chemistry of MDMA. *J. Psychoactive Drugs,* **18,** 291–304.

Shulgin, A. T. (1990). *History of MDMA.* In S. J. Peroutka, (Ed.). Ecstasy: The Clinical, Pharmacological and Neurotoxicological Effects of the Drug MDMA. Holland: Kluwer. 1–20.

Shulgin, A. T. and Nichols, D. E. (1978). *Characterization of three new psychotomimetics.* In R. Stillman and R. Willete (Eds.). The Psychopharmacology of Hallucinogens. New York: Pergamon Press, pp. 74–83.

Shulgin, A. and Shulgin, A. (1991). *PIHKAL*. Berkeley: Transform Press.

Slikker, W., Ali, S. F., Scallet, A. C., Frith, C. H., Newport, G. D. and Bailey, J. R. (1988). Neurochemical and neurohistological alterations in the rat and monkey produced by orally administered methylenedioxymethamphetamine (MDMA). *Toxicol. Appl. Pharmacol., 94,* 448–457.

Slikker, W. J., Holson, R. R., Ali, S. F., Kolta, M. G., Paule, M. G., Scallet, A. C., McMillan, D. E., Bailey, J. R., Hong, J. S. and Scalzo, R. M. (1989). Behavioral and neurochemical effects of orally administered MDMA in the rodent and nonhuman primate. *Neurotoxicol., 10,* 529–542.

Sprague, J. E. and Nichols, D. E. (1995). The monoamine oxidase-B inhibitor l-deprenyl protects against 3,4-methylenedioxymethamphetamine-induced lipid peroxidation and long-term serotonergic deficits. *J. Pharmacol. Exp. Ther., 273,* 667–673.

Sprague, J. E., Everman, S. L. and Nichols, D. E. (1998). An integrated hypothesis for the serotonergic axonal loss induced by 3,4-methylenedioxymethamphetamine. *Neurotoxicol., 19,* 427–442.

Suomi, S. J. (1999). *Attachment in rhesus monkeys.* In J. Cassidy and P. R. Shaver, (Eds.). Handbook of Attachment: Theory, Research and Clinical Applications. New York: Guilford Press, 181–197.

Sylvester, R. (1995). Ecstasy: the truth. *The Sunday Telegraph,* 19 Nov: 24.

Tancer, M. and Schuster, C. R. (1997). Serotonin and dopamine system interactions in the reinforcing properties of psychostimulants: a research strategy. *MAPS, 7*(3), 5–11.

Tancer, M. and Johanson, C. E. (1999). Subjective responses to MDMA and mCPP: A human dose run-up study. *CPDD,* 160.

Vollenweider, F., Gamma, A., Liechti, M. and Huber, T. (1998). Psychological and cardiovascular effects and short-term sequelae of MDMA (ecstasy) in MDMA-naïve healthy volunteers. *Neuropsychopharmacol., 19,* 241–251.

Vollenweider, F. X., Gamma, A., Liechti, M. and Huber, T. (1999). Is a single dose of MDMA harmless? *Neuropsychopharmacol., 21,* 598–600.

Watanabe, Y., Sakai, R. R., McEwen, B. S. and Mendelson, S. (1993). Stress and antidepressant effects on hippocampal and cortical 5-HT1A and 5-HT2 receptors and transport sites for serotonin. *Brain Res., 615,* 87–94.

Winstock, A. R. and King, L. A. (1996). Tablets often contain substances in addition to, or instead of, ecstasy, such as ketamine. *Lancet, 313,* 423–424.

Wolff, K., Hay, A. W. M., Sherlock, K. and Conner, M. (1996). Contents of "ecstasy." *Lancet, 346,* 1100–1101.

Young, F. (1986). *Opinion and recommended ruling, findings of fact, conclusions of law and decision of administrative law judge: submitted in the matter of MDMA scheduling.* U.S. Drug Enforcement Administration Docket no. 84–88.

Ziporyn, T. (1986). A growing industry and menace: makeshift laboratory's designer drugs. *JAMA,* **256,** 3061–3063.

Appendix C

Psychiatric Research with Hallucinogens: What Have We Learned?

Charles S. Grob, M.D.

PSYCHIATRIC RESEARCH with hallucinogens has resumed. After two decades of virtual prohibition, formal authorization from federal regulatory agencies to conduct investigative studies in the United States with these unique mind-altering substances has been successfully obtained (Strassman, 1991). The bitter and acrimonious debate that raged through the 1960s and 1970s and into the 1980s has largely subsided. Scientific and health policy makers have determined that these drugs, although possessing an inherent abuse potential, do have a safety profile of acceptable magnitude when compared to drugs currently the subject of formal research investigation as well as others actively dispensed in clinical practice. The U.S. Food and Drug Administration has therefore determined that formal and well-controlled investigations designed to assess the risk-benefit ratio of particular hallucinogenic substances may now be pursued. However, for such studies to proceed successfully and for the much heralded (and often vilified) potential of the hallucinogens to be explored, it is imperative that we fully grasp the lessons of the past. For, to paraphrase

Santayana, if we fail to understand our history, we will be condemned to repeat the patterns and reactions which will inevitably lead to yet another round of repudiation and rejection of this unique class of psychoactive substances, along with its inherent and inestimable potential for learning and healing.

Shamanistic Roots

Hallucinogens, throughout the breadth of time, have played a vital albeit hidden and mysterious role. They have often, in aboriginal and shamanic contexts, been at the absolute center of culture and world view (Dobkin de Rios, 1984). Opening up the doors to the spiritual planes, and accessing vital information imperative to tribal cohesion and survival, hallucinogenic plants became what some scholars have considered to be the bedrock of human civilization (Wasson, 1968; Wasson et al., 1978; Huxley, 1978). Within the context of shamanic society, these awe-inspiring botanicals were utilized to facilitate healing, divine the future, protect the community from danger and enhance learning (e.g. teaching hunters the ways of animals) (Cordova-Rios, 1971). However, with the advent of stratified and hierarchical societies, such plant potentiators came to be viewed as dangerous to the commonweal and controls were placed on direct and revelatory access to the sacred (Dobkin de Rios and Smith, 1976). In some societies (e.g. Aztec civilization) use of psychotropic plants was restricted to the select castes of the religious priesthood. In others, including the progenitors of our own contemporary Euro-American culture, absolute proscriptions on the use of plant drugs for divine purposes were decreed.

Repression of Shamanistic Traditions

To fully understand the enormous resistances to these drugs and the unique experiences they induce, it would be revealing to examine some elements of our historical legacy. A poorly appreciated period from fourteenth- through seventeenth-century European history has been the persecution of indigenous healers, predominantly women, during the reign of the Inquisition, particularly in Northern and Western Europe. During a span of three hundred years several million women were accused of practicing witchcraft and condemned to die. The Medieval scholar Jules Michelet has explored the complicity between ecclesiastical and medical authorities in the subjugation of non-sanctioned healing, commenting on the attitude of the Church "that if a woman dare cure without having studied, she is a witch and must die" (Michelet, 1965). To have "studied" in this context is to have faithfully adhered to the precepts and moral authority of the Church, and to have forsworn receiving knowledge from Nature.

A rich heritage of plant lore and applied healing had been passed down from pagan and pre-Christian Europe, rivaling and often surpassing the demonstrated efficacy of Church-sanctioned medical practitioners. Hallucinogenic plants with magical as well as healing properties were essential elements of this indigenous pharmacopoeia. Members of the *Solanaceae* family with their alkaloids atropine and scopolamine, including a great number of species of the genus Datura, as well as mandrake, henbane, and belladonna, had wide application as agents of healing and transcendence (Harner, 1973). In taking action against the indigenous use of psychotropic plants, the Church sought to eliminate a perceived threat to its oligarchic powers and reassert its monopoly on legitimate access to the supernatural (O'Neil, 1987). By casting the healer as a witch and the hallucinogenic plants as tools of Satan, the Church succeeded not only in eliminating competition to the elite physician class but also in virtually eradicating knowledge of these vestiges of pagan and shamanic consciousness.

A second historical period whose examination may be pertinent to understanding our ingrained cultural resistances and aversion to hallucinogens is the European conquest of the New World. Shortly after arrival in Central and South America in the late fifteenth and early sixteenth centuries, the invading Spanish Conquistadors observed an impressive array of psychoactive pharmacopoeia, including morning glory seeds (containing the potent hallucinogen, lysergic acid amide), peyote, and psilocybin mushrooms. These extraordinary plants were utilized by the native inhabitants to in-

duce an ecstatic intoxication and were an integral component of their aboriginal religion and ritual. As plant hallucinogens were attributed to have
supernatural powers, they were quickly perceived by the European invaders
as weapons of the Devil designed to prevent the triumph of Christianity
over traditional Indian religion (Furst, 1976). An early seventeenth-
century Spanish observer of native customs, Hernando Ruiz de Alarcon,
wrote of the idolatries he observed involving the consumption of the morning glory: "Olouihqui is a kind of seed-like lentils produced by a type of
vine in this land, which when drunk deprive of the senses, because it is
very powerful, and by this means they communicate with the devil, because he talks to them when they are deprived of judgment with the said
drink, and deceive them with different hallucinations, and they attribute it
to a god they say is inside the seed" (Guerra, 1971).

Identifying the threat not only to consolidating their power and control
over the conquered peoples, but also the danger of lower caste immigrant
Spaniards developing interest in native rituals and healing practices, The
Holy Inquisition of Mexico issued in 1616 a proclamation ordering the
persecution and excommunication of those who, under the influence of
"herbs and roots with which they lose and confound their senses, and the
illusions and fantastic representations they have, judge and proclaim after-
wards as revelation, or true notice of things to come . . ." (Guerra, 1967).
To continue to engage in native practices and utilize their traditional plant
hallucinogens as agents of knowledge and healing would risk indictment of
heresy and witchcraft, and inevitably the implementation of the crudest
punishments of the Inquisition, from public flogging to being burned alive
at the stake. Unable to accept the indigenous utilization of such psychoactive substances as anything other than idolatry and a threat to their
goals of domination and exploitation, the European conquerors denied
them legitimacy, endeavoring to expunge their traditions and knowledge.
Only by going deeply underground and maintaining their world view and
shamanic practices in secret from the dominant Euro-American culture,
has this knowledge survived.

Early Research with Hallucinogens

Interest in plant hallucinogens lay dormant until the second half of the nineteenth century when growing activities in the new fields of experimental physiology and pharmacology sparked efforts at laboratory analyses of medicinal plants. In the late 1880s German toxicologist Louis Lewin, often called the "father of modern psychopharmacology," received a collection of peyote samples from the Parke-Davis Pharmaceutical Company. Succeeding at isolating several alkaloids from the peyote, Lewin was unable to identify any of them as the psychoactive component through animal testing. The investigation was then taken up by Arthur Heffter, who characterized additional pure alkaloids from the cactus. By ingesting each of them he was able to identify the crucial one, which he named mescaline (Heffter, 1897).

Along with Lewin's published work, interest in plant hallucinogens was encouraged by increasing dissemination of knowledge of the Native American Indian use of peyote, a phenomenon of increasing prevalence as the century drew to a close. Obtaining a sample of peyote from the southwestern plains, physician and founder of the American Neurological Association Weir Mitchell conducted an experiment using himself as the subject. Although overwhelmed with the aesthetic power of the experience, describing that the peyote revealed "a certain sense of the things about me as having a more positive existence than usual," Mitchell expressed alarm that such a profound experience might not be successfully integrated within his contemporary context: "I predict a perilous reign of the mescal habit . . . The temptation to call again the enchanting magic of my experience will, I am sure, be too much for some men to resist after they have once set foot in this land of fairy colors where there seems so much to charm and so little to excite horror or disgust" (Mitchell, 1896).

Inspired by reports of Mitchell's self-experimentation, the prominent English physician Havelock Ellis decided to pursue a similar encounter with the plant hallucinogen, which he later reported as an experience of unparalleled magnitude, asserting that to "once or twice be admitted to the rites of mescal is not only an unforgettable delight but an educational influence of no mean value" (Ellis, 1897). Such unqualified praise of a drug with as yet no proven medical application, however, provoked harsh censure from the editors of the British Medical Journal who expressed grave concern of peyote's injurious potential and reprimanded Ellis for irresponsibly "putting the temptation before the section of the public which is always in search of new sensation" (British Medical Journal, 1898). Such a vituperative response to Ellis' naive efforts at publicizing and perhaps promoting auto-experimentation with magical plants is an early harbinger of the conflict that mired and paralyzed the field of hallucinogenic research some seventy years later.

Interest in the unusual psychogenic effects of peyote and, following its synthesis in 1919, mescaline, continued through the 1920s. Activities included further exploration of the unique visions induced by the drug by a variety of literary figures and scholars introduced to its exotic phenomena, although when William James experienced a severe gastro-intestinal reaction upon attempting to swallow a segment of peyote he is alleged to have stated: "Henceforth, I'll take the visions on trust" (Stevens, 1987). A comprehensive survey of the effects of mescaline was published by Karl Beringer, a close associate of Hermann Hesse and Carl Jung, in his massive tome "Der Meskalinrausch" (The Mescaline Inebriation) in 1927, followed a year later by Heinrich Kluver's Mescal: The "Divine" Plant and Its Psychological Effects, the first attempt at formal classification and analysis of mescaline visions (Kluver, 1928). And heralding the next phase of hallucinogen research, mescaline was touted by psychiatric researchers as a putative biochemical model for major mental disturbances, particularly schizophrenia (Guttman and Maclay, 1936; Stockings, 1940).

Dr. Hofmann's Serendipitous Discovery

The modern era of hallucinogen research began in the laboratory of Dr. Albert Hofmann, a senior research chemist for the Sandoz Pharmaceutical Company in Basel, Switzerland. In mid April 1943, Hofmann was engaged in work to chemically modify alkaloids from the rye ergot fungus, *Claviceps purpurea*, in an effort to develop a new analeptic agent (a respiratory stimulant). Acting on a premonition that earlier tests had missed something, he returned to and prepared a fresh batch of a compound he had previously synthesized in 1938, but which had proved at that time to have what were considered to be uninteresting results in animal testing. The chemical compound he had decided to return to after this five-year hiatus was the twenty-fifth in a series of lysergic acid amides, and had previously received the designation of LSD-25.

While working with a modest quantity of this compound for further study, Hofmann complained of restlessness and feeling dizzy and decided to return to his home to rest. He subsequently would write that upon reaching home and lying down with his eyes closed he experienced an "extreme activity of the imagination . . . there surged upon me an uninterrupted stream of fantastic images of extraordinary plasticity and vividness and accompanied by an intense kaleidoscope-like play of colors. After about two hours, the not unpleasant inebriation, which had been experienced while I was fully conscious, disappeared" (Hofmann, 1983).

Concluding that he had probably accidentally absorbed a small quantity of the compound through his skin, Hofmann set out three days later, on April 19, 1943, to replicate the, phenomena by self administering what he considered to be an extremely small and cautious dose, 250 micrograms. Intending to record his subjective experiences of what he had assumed to be a very low dose of the peculiar substance, less than an hour later Hofmann began to feel the onset of what was to be a powerful and indeed frightening altered state of consciousness, and again felt compelled to return to his home. Hofmann would later report "On the way home, my condition began to assume threatening forms . . . Everything in my field of vision wavered and was distorted as if seen in a curved mirror. I also had the sensation of being unable to move from the spot. Nevertheless, my assistant later told me that we had traveled very rapidly . . . My surroundings had now transformed themselves in more terrifying ways. Everything in the room spun around, and the familiar objects and pieces of furniture assumed grotesque, threatening forms. They were in continuous motion, animated, as if driven by an inner restlessness . . . Even worse than these demonic transformations of the outer world, were the alterations that I perceived in myself, in my inner being. Every exertion of my will, every attempt to put an end to the disintegrations of the outer world and the dissolution of my ego, seemed to be wasted effort. A demon had invaded me, had taken possession of my body, mind and soul." Shortly thereafter, Hofmann would describe, "the climax of my despondent condition had passed . . . the horror softened and gave way to a feeling of good fortune and gratitude . . . now, little by little I could begin to enjoy the unprecedented colors and plays of shapes that persisted behind my closed eyes. Kaleidoscopic, fantastic images surged in on me, alternating, variegated, opening and then closing themselves in circles and spirals, exploding in colored fountains . . . Exhausted, I then slept, to awake next morning refreshed, with a clear head, though still somewhat tired physically. A sensation of well-being and renewed life flowed through me" (Hofmann, 1983). Dr. Hofmann's shocking experience of madness and transcendence, precipitated by an infinitesimally low dose of what would soon be recognized as the most potent psychoactive substance known to man, heralded the advent of a new era of psychiatric research committed to uncovering the mysteries of the mind and revealing the basis of mental illness.

The Psychotomimetic Model

Albert Hofmann's discovery of LSD soon led to a period of intense interest and activity designed to explore its utility as a model of understanding and treating psychotic illness. Such a direction was consistent with earlier investigations equating the mescaline catalyzed altered state of consciousness with the subjective experience of schizophrenic patients (Guttman and Maclay, 1936; Stockings, 1940). Tayleur Stockings had described the similarities between the two states: "Mescaline intoxication is indeed a true 'schizophrenia' if we use the word in its literal sense of 'split mind,' for the characteristic effect of mescaline is a molecular fragmentation of the entire personality, exactly similar to that found in schizophrenic patients . . . Thus the subject of the mescaline psychosis may believe that he has become transformed into some great personage, such as a god or a legendary character, or a being from another world. This is a well-known symptom found in states such as paraphrenia and paranoia" (Stockings, 1940). Noting the enormity of perceptual disturbances induced by LSD, coupled with the sensation in some subjects of losing their mind, as had transiently been the case with Dr. Hofmann, Sandoz Pharmaceutical in 1947 began actively marketing LSD to psychiatric researchers and practitioners as a tool for understanding psychoses. Not only was LSD experimentation in normal subjects proposed as a viable model for studying the pathogenesis of psychotic illness, but psychiatrists were encouraged to self-administer the drug so as to gain insight into the subjective world of the patient with serious mental illness (Stevens, 1987). For a young field struggling to gain credibility as a medical science, this model of chemically controlled psychosis emerged as a propitious sign for the future.

Preoccupation with the hallucinogen-induced psychotomimetic model continued through the 1950s. The psychotomimetic position was summarized by one its leading proponents, Harvard psychiatrist Max Rinkel: "The psychotic phenomena produced were predominantly schizophrenia-like symptoms, manifested in disturbances of thought and speech, changes in affect and mood, changes in perception, production of hallucinations and delusions, depersonalizations and changes in behavior. Rorschach tests and concrete-abstract thinking tests showed responses quite similar to those obtained with schizophrenics" (Rinkel and Denber, 1958). It became increasingly apparent, however, that although an impressive array of psychiatric researchers and theoreticians had elucidated and elaborated upon the startling degree of resemblance between schizophrenia and the hallucinogenic experience, a growing consensus was emerging that the dissimilarities between the two states essentially obviated the value of the chemical psychosis model (Grinspoon and Bakalar, 1979). Speaking at the First International Congress of Neuropsychopharmacology in 1959, the legendary Manfred Bleuler enunciated the central argument in opposition to the psychotomimetic model. He stated that it was the gradual and inexorable progression of a symptom complex that included disturbed thought processes, depersonalization and auditory hallucinations, evolving into a generalized functional incapacitation that was characteristic of schizophrenia. He concluded with the demonstrative declaration that although the psychotomimetic drugs may have strengthened our conceptual understanding of organic psychoses, they have "contributed nothing to the understanding of the pathogenesis of schizophrenia" (Bleuler, 1959).

Hallucinogen Research and the Role of the CIA

Following the end of World War II, as relations with our former ally the Soviet Union began to deteriorate and Cold War tensions heightened, a program was initiated by the U.S. Central Intelligence Agency to develop a speech-inducing drug for use in interrogations of suspected enemy agents. Such a search was in part stimulated by knowledge of prior, albeit unsuccessful, efforts by Nazi medical researchers at the Dachau Concentration Camp to utilize mescaline as an agent of mind control (Marks, 1979). By the early 1950s the CIA had acquired from Sandoz Pharmaceutical a large quantity of the highly touted psychotomimetic, LSD, and had begun their own extensive testing program. Early experiments often involved the furtive "dosing" of unwitting subjects, including employees of the CIA and other intelligence organizations, soldiers and customers solicited by prostitutes in the service of the CIA. Given the ill-prepared mental set of the victim, the often adverse setting in which the "experiment" occurred, and the lack of therapeutic aftercare, it is no surprise that highly deleterious outcomes, including suicide, did occur. Although knowledge of this irresponsible and ethically suspect association between the CIA and hallucinogenic substances remained suppressed for the next twenty years, knowledge of such activities was ultimately obtained through the Freedom of Information Act (Marks, 1979; Lee and Schlain, 1985).

Through the 1950s, as Cold War fears escalated, the CIA began to develop an affinity for the psychotomimetic model then in vogue. In order to further their own goals of investigating the mind-control potentials of hallucinogenic drugs, the CIA began to recruit and fund a number of distinguished psychiatric researchers. Included among these was Ewen Cameron, elected President of the American Psychiatric Association in 1953 and first President of the World Psychiatric Association. Capitalizing on the

CIA's preoccupation with LSD's purported ability to break down familiar behavior patterns, Cameron received funding to develop a bizarre and unorthodox method for treating severe mental illness. The treatment protocol began with "sleep therapy," where patients were sedated with barbiturates for a several-month period, and was followed by a "depatterning" phase of massive electroshock and frequent doses of LSD designed to obliterate past behavior patterns. Patients were then once again heavily sedated, and subsequently subjected to a prolonged "psychic driving" reconditioning phase where they received constant auditory bombardment from speakers under their pillows repeating tape-recorded messages, with some patients hearing the same message repeated a quarter of a million times. Given the gross excesses in all modalities of this "treatment," inevitably severe neuropsychiatric deterioration was incurred by many of Cameron's unconsented subjects (Marks, 1979; Lee and Schlain, 1985). Ultimately, the efforts of the CIA and their contract psychiatrists came to naught as their ill-advised collaboration with hallucinogens yielded little of value to support either the CIA's mind-control theories or the psychotomimetic investigations of psychiatric researchers.

The Psycholytic Treatment Model

Early experimentation in Switzerland following Albert Hofmann's discovery in the 1940s had discerned a phenomena quite different than that of the much heralded yet bizarre psychotomimetic mental experience. In subjects given a relatively low dose of LSD, there appeared to occur a release of repressed psychic material, particularly in anxiety states and obsessional neuroses. By allowing this otherwise repressed and threatening material to flow effortlessly into consciousness, investigators surmised that low-dose LSD treatment could facilitate the psychotherapy process (Stoll, 1947). Application of the low-dose model in Europe as well as the United States ascertained that psycholytic treatment had particular value with patients with rigid defense mechanisms and excessively strict superego structures. By facilitating ego regression, uncovering early childhood memories, and inducing an affective release, psychiatrists claimed to have achieved a breakthrough in reducing the duration and improving the outcome of psychotherapeutic treatment (Chandler and Hartmann, 1960). Problems arose with the psycholytic paradigm, however, as critics noted that the content of regressed material released from the unconscious was extremely sensitive to the psychiatrist's own analytic orientation, in most cases Freudian or Jungian. Questions arose over whether the phenomena observed in the psychotherapeutic sessions, including the often positive treatment outcome, were not simply attributable to the presence of heightened powers of suggestibility. Moreover, with psycholytic treatments, care had to be taken to utilize sufficiently low dosages of the hallucinogen that the patient's ego would not be overwhelmed to the point where verbal analysis would be inhibited. When in the course of psycholytic psychotherapy higher dosages were utilized, the resultant experience could no longer be contained within the intended theoretical framework, thus necessitating delineation of an entirely new paradigm.

The Psychedelic Treatment Model

Psychiatrists utilizing the higher dose model on their patients, as well as self-experimenting on themselves, quickly realized that they had accessed an entirely new and novel dimension of consciousness. As Dr. Hofmann had experienced during his own exploration, this unexpected level of awareness could alternately be rapturous or terrifying. The first psychiatrist to explore this paradigm was the Canadian researcher Humphry Osmond. Utilizing first mescaline, and later LSD, Osmond devoted his studies to the treatment of alcoholism, a notoriously difficult and refractory condition. Noting that some alcoholics were only able to cease their pathological drinking behaviors after they had experienced a terrifying, hallucinatory episode of delirium tremens during alcohol withdrawal, Osmond set out to replicate this state through utilization of a high dose hallucinogen model. Observing that what distinguished his treatment successes from his treatment failures was whether a transcendent and mystical state of consciousness was attained, Osmond recognized the strong resemblance to states of religious conversion, bringing to mind William

James' old axiom that "the best cure for dipsomania is religiomania." Dissatisfied with the prevailing jargon, and arguing that his model demonstrated that hallucinogens did much more than "mimic psychosis," Osmond introduced at the 1957 meeting of the New York Academy of Sciences the term psychedelic, explaining that the "mind manifesting" state did not necessarily produce a predictable and pathological sequence of events, but rather could catalyze an enriching and life-changing vision. And in presaging the cacophonous debate that would shortly fall upon the infant field of hallucinogen research, Osmond concluded that the psychedelic model not only allowed us to escape "Freud's gloomier moods that persuaded him that a happy man is a self-deceiver," but would soon come to the aid of humanity's imperiled existence and "have a part to play in our survival as a species" (Osmond, 1957).

The Prohibition of Hallucinogen Research

With the evolution to the psychedelic model, hallucinogens moved beyond the bounds of control of the medical elite (Neill, 1987). No longer could they be confined to investigations of a model psychosis, nor could they be contained within the framework of conventional psychiatric therapies with implicit prescribed roles for doctor and patient. By blurring the boundaries between religion and science, between sickness and health, and between healer and sufferer, the psychedelic model entered the realm of applied mysticism. As word of the astounding phenomenon induced by the psychedelic model spread into the culture at large, the inevitable backlash occurred. Horrified that this extraordinary investigative probe had been appropriated from their control, the leaders of the psychiatric profession directed harsh criticism at their irrepressible and increasingly evangelistic colleagues. Roy Grinker, the first editor of the prestigious Archives of General Psychiatry, in a 1963 editorial castigated those psychiatric researchers who had become preoccupied with administering "the drug to themselves, and some, who became enamored with the mystical hallucinatory state, eventually in their 'mystique' became unqualified as competent investigators" (Grinker, 1963). And a year later, in the Journal of the

American Medical Association, Grinker charged researchers with "using uncontrolled, unscientific methods. In fact, these professionals are widely known to participate in drug ingestion, rendering their conclusions biased by their own ecstasy . . . The psychotomimetics are being 'bootlegged,' and as drugs now under scientific investigation they are being misused" (Grinker, 1964). In moving beyond the boundaries of conventional scientific inquiry, the hallucinogens had "become invested with an aura of magic" (Cole and Katz, 1964), and thus could no longer be provided the status and protection of their elite profession. The covenant had been broken. The hallucinogens, along with the proponents of their continued exploration, were cast out, becoming pariahs in a land and a time that increasingly viewed them as threats to public safety and social order.

By the mid-1960s, the secret was out. Growing interest in hallucinogens had catalyzed, and was catalyzed by, profound cultural shifts. Along with the social upheaval surrounding opposition to an increasingly unpopular war in Southeast Asia, hallucinogens assumed a central role in a movement that began to question many of the basic values and precepts of mainstream Euro-American culture. The populace, fueled by sensational media accounts, grew to identify hallucinogens as a prime suspect in inciting the accelerating state of cultural havoc. Along with the drugs themselves, adherents of the experimental and treatment models became increasingly identified as part of the problem. Such circumstances were in no way improved by the rash pronouncements from the radical wing of what had rapidly become identified as an hallucinogen-inspired political movement. The leaders of one notorious research group in particular drew public ire and aroused anxiety and panic by such proclamations as: "Make no mistake: the effect of consciousness-expanding drugs will be to transform our concepts of human nature, of human potentialities, of existence. The game is about to be changed, ladies and gentleman . . . These possibilities naturally threaten every branch of the Establishment. The dangers of external change appear to frighten us less than the peril of internal change. LSD is more frightening than the Bomb!" (Leary and Alpert, 1962).

In response to escalating fears that hallucinogens had become an out-of-control menace to public safety and cultural stability, the government moved to restrict access to these potent agents of change. Psychiatric leaders, gravely concerned by the threat to public mental health, and perhaps to their professional image as well, vehemently urged government regulating agencies to tighten their controls. Roy Grinker, illustrious psychiatrist and President of the American Medical Association, issued an urgent warning to his colleagues that greater damage lay ahead unless usage of these hazardous chemical agents was contained. Going beyond merely calling for the psychiatry profession to take action against this growing peril, which would include denouncing the renegades within its own ranks, Grinker castigated the government for having been woefully lacking in vigilance and having neglected its duty: "The Food and Drug Administration has failed in its policing functions. The drugs are indeed dangerous even when used under the best of precautions and conditions" (Grinker, 1964).

Driven into action by increasingly lurid media and law enforcement accounts of widespread hallucinogen use among the young, amidst dire warnings that this insidious threat would erode the values and work ethic of future generations, government regulators had no choice but to act. In 1965 the Congress passed the Drug Abuse Control Amendment, which placed tight restrictions on hallucinogen research, forcing all research applications to be routed through the FDA for approval. In April, 1966, succumbing to mounting adverse publicity, Sandoz Pharmaceuticals ceased the marketing of what their esteemed research chemist Albert Hofmann would come to call "my problem child" (Hoffman, 1983). Also during the spring of 1966, Senator Robert Kennedy called for Congressional Hearings on the problem. Kennedy, whose wife Ethel had reportedly received psychiatric treatments with LSD, expressed concern that potentially vital research was being obstructed, questioning: "Why if they were worthwhile six months ago, why aren't they worthwhile now? . . . I think we have given too much emphasis and so much attention to the fact that it can be dangerous and that it can hurt an individual who uses it . . . that perhaps to some extent we have lost sight of the fact that it can be very, very helpful in our society if used properly" (Lee and Schlain, 1985). Kennedy's pleas went unheeded, as over the next few years more and more stringent restrictions were imposed on hallucinogen research, culminating in the Bu-

reau of Narcotics and Dangerous Drugs (the predecessor to the Drug Enforcement Agency) decision to place the hallucinogens in the Schedule I
class, reserved for dangerous drugs of abuse with no medical value. Research ground to a virtual halt. Government, civic and medical leaders had
all responded to their call to duty, permanently expunging, they hoped,
what President Lyndon Johnson had declared in his State of the Union address in January, 1968, "these powders and pills which threaten our nation's health, vitality and self-respect" (Stevens, 1987).

Discounting Hallucinogen Research

Hallucinogens, in the guise of an experimental probe into the mysterious world of mental illness, had burst on the scene during the infancy of
psychiatric research. They had not only unleashed a firestorm of controversy as a highly touted therapeutic intervention, but had greatly contributed
to the development of the exciting new specialty of laboratory neurochemistry research. Access to these unique agents for animal research has been permitted to continue unimpeded, and they have contributed greatly to our
understanding of neurotransmitter systems, brain-imaging techniques and
behavioral pharmacology (Jacobs, 1984; Freedman, 1986). And yet, human
research with hallucinogens had, until now, vanished from the scene. Discounted for ever having held value or potential, it is as if they had never been
with us. A source of embarrassment and shame, hallucinogen research became a non-issue, virtually disappearing from the professional literature and
educational curriculums. By the early 1970s, psychiatric researchers and
academicians had perceived that to continue to advocate for human research with hallucinogens, or even to be identified with past interest in their
therapeutic potential, might seriously jeopardize their future careers. Difficult decisions had to be made. From the mid 1960s onward, a split began to
appear in the ranks of psychiatric hallucinogen researchers. For those who
would maintain their enthusiasm for the potentials of these singular substances, a path of professional marginalization would follow. For those who
would take a stand against their perfidious threat, accolades and professional
advancement would be forthcoming. For most, however, it was to be a

process of quietly disengaging, often from what had been a passionate interest, and redirecting their careers toward tamer and less disputable areas. With very few exceptions (Grinspoon and Bakalar, 1979; Grinspoon and Bakalar, 1986; Strassman, 1984), a veil of silence had descended over the putative role of hallucinogen research in psychiatry.

The Future of Hallucinogen Research in Psychiatry

Where are we to go with this most unusual class of psychoactive substances? Some would say it is best to let sleeping dogs lie, that the hallucinogens only brought discord and controversy to the ranks of psychiatry and their re-examination can only lead to further turmoil and acrimony. Psychiatry has moved far beyond the time where hallucinogens were viewed as being on the cutting edge of research investigation. Many psychiatrists graduating from training programs in the last decade are not even aware of the role hallucinogens once did play in the arena of legitimate research. The conventional point of view is that these drugs are potential substances of abuse, nothing more. Within mainstream, academic psychiatry forums for discussion of the relative merits of resuming inquiries into this area have been restricted. What was once a roar of often vituperative debate has receded to barely a whisper.

Perhaps this twenty-five-year period of quiescence and retreat into relative obscurity has been necessary to finally give the question of hallucinogens a fair hearing. We have seen in a prior epoch of investigation a playing field painfully polarized between ardent advocates and fervent foes of the hallucinogens' putative role as agents of discovery and healing. The truth has always rested somewhere in between the dichotomous poles of panacea and toxin. The protagonists of the past, whose careers and integrity so often appeared to be interwoven with the content and outcome of their fierce debate, are exiting the arena. Rumblings of renewed interest are being heard within the halls of academic psychiatry. A new dialogue is slowly starting to emerge. Hopefully, the lessons of the past will be appreciated, and utilized to forge a partnership and collaboration where divergent perspectives will be given a fair and open hearing, and the true potential of the hallucinogens may finally be illuminated.

As the sleeping giant of hallucinogen research emerges from its twenty-five-year slumber, it will perceive that the world of psychiatry has vastly changed from when it was put to rest. The once reigning rulers of psychoanalysis have receded to positions of relative obscurity as the field has become progressively dominated by the adherents of biological reductionism. The insights gleaned from the individual case study, once the standard of psychoanalytic investigation, have been devalued and supplanted by the rigorous methodological research design of modern psychiatry. In the future, the putative value of hallucinogens in psychiatry can no longer rest on claims deriving from anecdotal case studies, as inspiring as they may be, but rather must evolve out of the findings of well-structured, controlled, scientific investigation. To achieve relevance and be accepted as a reputable field of study, hallucinogen research must satisfy the standards of contemporary psychiatric research. To maintain an iconoclastic insistence that the very nature of these substances transcends standard research designs would be to prolong their marginalization and deny the opportunity finally to explore their potential utility.

The knowledge base of biological psychiatry and the neurosciences has exploded over the last two decades, facilitated in part by probes and techniques developed with hallucinogen research in animals (Jacobs, 1984; Freedman, 1986). The potential for further advances in our understanding of the mechanisms of brain function has been recognized and enunciated at a technical meeting of the National Institute on Drug Abuse (NIDA) in July, 1992, that concluded that it is now time to move beyond pure animal research into the realm of human investigation. We are now on the threshold of initiating studies utilizing state-of-the-art research techniques, including sophisticated brain-imaging scans, neuroendocrine challenge tests, and receptor-binding studies in human subjects. The strategy of pursuing such biological investigations will likely not only yield valuable new information in the neurosciences, but facilitate the relegitimization of human research with hallucinogens and ultimately become a prelude to the re-exploration of their effects on perception, cognition, and emotion.

One of the most controversial arenas of hallucinogen research during the 1950s and 1960s, and persisting as an alluring hope, has been their putative role in alleviating mental suffering. During a mere fifteen-year period, over a thousand clinical papers were published in the professional literature discussing the experiences of 40,000 patients treated with hallucinogens (Grinspoon and Bakalar, 1979). While many of these reports were presented in the form of descriptive case studies and are attributed little value by contemporary research standards, they can help point the way for future investigations. A wide variety of psychopathological phenomena were subjected to intervention with hallucinogens, often leading to encouraging reports of positive clinical outcomes. Unfortunately, examining these stimulating accounts in retrospect reveals notable flaws in their design, including primitive and by today's standards deficient measures designed to evaluate therapeutic change, lack of outcome follow-up and unwillingness to utilize appropriate control subjects. As the debate over hallucinogens intensified, it also became apparent that from both warring camps investigators' biases (whether conscious or unconscious) were confounding their results. From our current vantage point, it is often difficult to ascertain the true significance of this past research other than to appreciate that sufficient clinical change appears to have been catalyzed that further investigation is merited. And as we prepare to delve into the question of the hallucinogens' application to treatment models, it will be essential that we control for the flaws that made a previous generation of research suspect. State-of-the-art research methodology must be utilized, including proper attention to set and setting, control populations and measures of short- and long-term treatment outcome. An atmosphere of active collaboration among investigators with contrasting perspectives needs to be established, avoiding at all costs the schism which led to the collapse of earlier efforts.

The Relevance of the Past

We are on the threshold of initiating explorations which may have considerable ramifications for our future. There is much at stake and much to learn. But in order to take full advantage of this opportunity we must fully understand our past, including that which we know from cultures distant to our own place and time. Plant-derived hallucinogens once played a vital, albeit poorly appreciated role in our prehistorical lineage (Furst, 1976; Dobkin de Rios, 1984). While psychiatry has traditionally held a disparaging and pathologizing view toward shamanic belief systems and practices (Devereux, 1958), evidence supplied by transcultural anthropological investigators (Jilek, 1971; Noll, 1983) demonstrates that shamanic practices may actually be conducive to high levels of psychological health and functioning. To move beyond the commonly held psychiatric viewpoint that shamanism is nothing more than primitivism and the prehistorical well-spring of mental illness, would allow for receptivity to learning from a paradigm that has incorporated for thousands of years the utilization of hallucinogens as a vital facet of belief systems and healing practices (Bravo and Grob, 1989). If we are to assess optimally the true clinical efficacy and safety of the hallucinogens, it is imperative that we be conscious of the critical extrapharmacological variables that we know to be integral to the shamanic model. Ample attention and sensitivity must be given to the preparation for the hallucinogen experience, the powerful expectation effects directed toward predetermined therapeutic goals, the formalized structure of the session and the integration of the altered-state experience in the days, weeks and months following the experience. The failure to adhere to any of these aspects of the shamanic paradigm would be to deny hallucinogen research the full opportunity to test its true value.

What removes the shamanic world view so far from our own, and consequently presents the greatest challenges when attempting to incorporate its insights into contemporary research methodology, is the belief that the plant hallucinogens are sacraments of divine origin. However, it is this reverential and spiritual utilization of psychoactive substances that so pointedly distinguishes the practices of tribal and shamanic peoples from our own contemporary profaned and pathologized context of drug abuse. Hallucinogens in the shamanic world have traditionally played a critical role in rites of initiation, providing personal regeneration and radical change, and are perceived as essential to the process of growth and maturity and the acquisition of meaning (Grob and Dobkin de Rios, 1992; Zoja, 1989). They are not misused or abused, and are not agents of societal chaos and destruction. Their use is fully sanctioned and integrated into the mainstream of society, and commonly utilized in ritually prescribed and elder-facilitated ceremonies. The hypersuggestible properties of the hallucinogens, utilized within a highly controlled set and setting, achieves a powerful effect, reinforcing cultural cohesion and commitment. These apparent beneficial effects of shamanic hallucinogen use contrast markedly with the destructive outcomes often observed in our own contemporary contexts (Dobkin de Rios and Grob, 1993).

An Illustrative Model

One of the most exciting areas of investigation from the past era of hallucinogen research was the treatment of severe, refractory alcoholism. In the 1950s psychiatric researchers had identified the similarities between the spectrum of the LSD experience and the phenomenology of delirium tremens (Osmond, 1957; Ditman and Whittlesey, 1959). As alcoholism was notorious for its lack of responsiveness to conventional treatment approaches, great interest and energies were directed towards this area of study. Highly impressive short-term results of treatment with hallucinogens (Chwelos et al., 1959; MacLean et al., 1961; Van Dusen et al., 1967) gave impetus to a surge of enthusiasm that a dramatic and effective intervention had finally been found. Additional support was forthcoming from Bill Wilson, the founder of Alcoholics Anonymous, who revealed that his own carefully supervised experiences with LSD had not only been a highly valuable personal experience, but were also fully compatible with the tenets of the movement he had started (Grof, 1987). However, as the level of discord within the psychiatric profession and the degree of alarm in the public heightened, resistance to accepting the hallucinogen model for alcoholism intensified. As mainstream psychiatry could no longer stand idly by in the face of threatened radical upheaval, so the Board of Trustees of Alcoholics Anonymous felt compelled to reject their creator Bill Wilson's proposed endorsement.

It soon became apparent that the methodological shortcomings of the research alleging to demonstrate unequivocally positive results in the treatment of alcoholism would undermine progress in the field. Poorly controlled research design, with questionable measures of change and inadequate follow-up led to charges that hallucinogen advocates had been blinded by their own enthusiasm and had misinterpreted and misrepresented their findings. Opponents of the hallucinogen treatment model would subsequently conduct their own clinical trials, designed to refute what they perceived as dangerous and exaggerated claims of therapeutic success (Smart et al., 1966; Hollister et al., 1969; Ludwig, Levine and Stark, 1970). These studies, which purported to demonstrate an entire lack of treatment efficacy of models utilizing hallucinogens, were received by the psychiatric establishment with great relief. In fact, the Ludwig, Levine and Stark study provided such reassurance to a profession so shaken by its own iconoclasts, as well as satisfying contemporary formal medical research standards with such aplomb, that it was awarded the prestigious Lester N. Hofheimer Prize for Research from the American Psychiatric Association.

Nevertheless, the investigations designed to provide the last word on the "failed" hallucinogen treatment model have themselves come under scathing attack. Not only have the investigators' lack of appreciation of set and setting, failure to adequately prepare their patients for the experience and refusal to allow for follow-up integration been identified (Grinspoon and Bakalar, 1979), but the capricious nature of medical research has itself been implicated. "At a time when LSD was popular, Levine and Ludwig (1967) had reported positive results . . . When LSD fell out of favor and the positive results became politically unwise, they obtained negative results. Unconsciously or consciously they built into their study a number of antitherapeutic elements that guaranteed a therapeutic failure" (Grof, 1980).

The discussion of the potential role of hallucinogens in the treatment of alcoholism, and by inference its application to other psychiatric disorders as well, would not be complete without an examination of the role of the plant hallucinogen, peyote, in the treatment of Native American Indians.

Evidence exists that peyote was in widespread use in Central America and revered as a medicine and religious sacrament as early as 200 B.C. (Furst, 1976). After the American Civil War, the use of peyote moved north of the Rio Grande River and quickly spread to dozens of native tribes throughout the United States and Canada. During the 1870s and 1880s a peyote vision religion developed in reaction to the inexorable encroachment of nonnative peoples onto the Indian lands and the associated, deliberate destruction of native culture. With the defeat and subjugation of the Native American people, alcoholism became epidemic. Although until recently faced with unrelenting political repression by the U.S. government, the Native American Church, a syncretistic church combining elements of traditional Indian religion and Christianity and utilizing peyote as its ritual sacrament, has been recognized by anthropologists and psychiatrists as being the only effective treatment for endemic alcoholism (Schultes, 1938; La Barre, 1947; Bergman, 1971; Albaugh and Anderson, 1974). Karl Menninger, a revered figure in the development of American Psychiatry in the twentieth century, has stated: "Peyote is not harmful to these people; it is beneficial, comforting, inspiring, and appears to be spiritually nourishing. It is a better antidote to alcohol than anything the missionaries, the white man, the American Medical Association, and the public health services have come up with" (Bergman, 1971).

Integral to the positive treatment outcome with peyote has been its sacramental utilization within the ritual context of mystical-religious experience. The Native American Church is a clear contemporary example of the successful application of the shamanic model to the treatment of severe, refractory illness. Although the Native American Church applies to a circumscribed and relatively homogenous population, it provides a valuable lesson on the importance of the shamanic model and the need for attentiveness to set and setting, intention, preparation and integration, as well as group identification. If we are to develop optimal research designs for evaluating the therapeutic utility of hallucinogens, it will not be sufficient to adhere to strict standards of scientific methodology alone. We must also pay heed to the examples provided us by such successful applications of the shamanic paradigm. It will only be then, when we have wedded our state-of-the-art research designs to the wisdom accrued from the past, that we will adequately appreciate what role hallucinogens may have in our future.

Conclusion

After a twenty-five-year period of virtual prohibition, formal psychiatric research with hallucinogenic drugs has resumed. This article has reviewed the process by which hallucinogens came to be viewed as beyond the pale of respected and sanctioned clinical investigation, and has directed attention to the importance of fully understanding the lessons of the past so as to avoid a similar fate for recently approved research endeavors. The shamanistic use of hallucinogenic plants as agents designed to facilitate healing, acquire knowledge and enhance societal cohesion were brutally repressed in both the Old and New Worlds by the progenitors of our own contemporary Euro-American culture, often with complicity of the medical professions. Knowledge of the properties and potentials of these consciousness-altering plants was forgotten or driven deeply underground for centuries. It was not until the late 1800s that German pharmaceutical researchers investigating the properties of peyote rediscovered the profound and highly unusual effects of these substances. A dispute anticipating the virulent controversies of the 1960s ensued, however, pitting proponents of this new model of consciousness exploration against those who questioned the propriety of their colleagues enthusiasm for self-experimentation and penchant for sweeping proclamations. The history of hallucinogen research in the twentieth century has revolved around this regrettable polarization, and as such has impeded the evolution of the field.

Developments in the second half of the twentieth century were catalyzed by the remarkable discoveries of the Swiss research chemist, Albert Hofmann. In the wake of his synthesis of the extraordinarily potent psychoactive substance, lysergic acid diethylamide, a period of active investigation ensued. Notable gains were accomplished utilizing the psychotomimetic model for understanding mental illness and the low-dose psycholytic approach for the treatment of a variety of psychiatric conditions. It soon became apparent, however, that these models possessed inherent limitations when applied to the orthodox psychiatric constructs then in vogue. The implementation of the high-dose psychedelic model, in spite of its apparent utility in treating resistant conditions such as refractory alcoholism, presented even greater difficulties in conforming to the boundaries of conventional theory and practice. Acceptance of hallucinogens as reputable tools for investigation and agents for treatment were dealt a further and near fatal blow when they became embroiled in the cultural wars of the 1960s. Together with revelations of unethical activities of psychiatric researchers under contract to military intelligence and the CIA, the highly publicized and controversial behaviors of hallucinogen enthusiasts led to the repression of efforts to investigate formally these substances. For the next twenty-five years, research with hallucinogens assumed pariah status within academic psychiatry, virtually putting an end to formal dialogue and debate.

We now have before us the opportunity to resurrect the long dormant field of hallucinogen research. However, if the debacle of the past is to be avoided, it is imperative that we learn from the lessons of prior generations of researchers who saw their hopes and accomplishments dissipate under the pressures of cultural apprehension and the threat of professional ostracism. It is essential that the mistakes of the past not be replicated. Definitive steps to end the protracted period of silence and inactivity have been initiated. Contemporary investigators will need to proceed tactfully however, and with respect for the anxieties that this work may provoke in their colleagues. Serious effort must be taken to facilitate active dialogue and collaboration. Current and accepted models of research design must be rigorously adhered to, for to disregard the state of contemporary scientific investigation would ultimately undermine the goals of fully exploring the rich potential of these substances. It will also be critical to learn from the wisdom accrued over the ages in cultures with world views quite different from our own. Although much of the knowledge of the shamanic utilization of plant hallucinogens has been lost with the passage of time, investigators must appreciate the vital role that set and setting have on determining outcome, and incorporate such parameters in their research designs. An opening now exists to explore this fascinating yet poorly understood class of psychoactive substances. Whether we can successfully take advantage of this opportunity will depend ultimately on how well we have learned the lessons of the past.

References

Albaugh, BJ (1974) Peyote in the treatment of alcoholism among American Indians. *Am J Psychiatry* 131, 1247–1250.

Bergman, RL (1971) Navajo peyote use: Its apparent safety. *Amer J Psychiatry* 128, 695–699.

Berringer, K (1927) *Der Mescalinrausch.* Springer, Berlin.

Bleuler, M (1958) Comparison of drug-induced and endogenous psychoses in man. In PB Breatly, R Deniker, Raduco-Thomas, D (Eds): *Proceedings of the First International Congress of Neuropsychopharmacology.* Elsevier, Amsterdam.

Bravo, G, Grob, C (1989) Shamans, sacraments and psychiatrists. *J Psychoactive Drugs* 21,123–128.

Chandler, AL, Hartman, MA (1960) Lysergic acid diethylamide (LSD-25) as a facilitating agent in psychotherapy. *Arch Gen Psychiatry* 2, 286–299.

Chwelos, N, Blewett, DB, Smith, CM, Hoffer, A (1959) Use of d-lysergic acid diethylamide in the treatment of alcoholism. *Quarterly J Studies Alcohol* 20, 577–590.

Cole, JO, Katz, M (1964) The psychotomimetic drugs. *JAMA* 187, 182–185.

Cordova-Rios, M (1971) *The Wizard of the Upper Amazon.* Atheneum, New York.

De Rios, MD, Smith, DE (1976) Using or abusing? An anthropological approach to the study of psychoactive drugs. *J Psychedel Drugs* 8, 263–266.

De Rios, MD, Grob, CS (1993) Hallucinogens, suggestibility and adolescence in cross-cultural perspective. *Yearbook of Ethnomedicine 3,* 113–132.

Devereux, G (1958) Cultural thought models in primitive and modern psychiatric theories. *Psychiatry* 21, 359–374.

Ditman, KS, Whittlesey, JRB (1959) Comparisons of the LSD experience and delirium tremens. *Arch Gen Psychiatry* 1, 47.

Ellis, H (1897) Mescal: A new artificial paradise. *Annual Report of the Smithsonian Institution,* pp. 537–548.

Freedman, DX (1986) Hallucinogenic drug research—if so, so what?: Symposium summary and commentary. *Pharmacol Biochem Behav*: 24, 407–415.

Furst-PT (1976) *Hallucinogens and Culture*. Chandler and Sharp, Novato, CA.

Grinker, R (1963) Lysergic acid diethylamide. *Arch Gen Psychiatry* 8, 425.

Grinker, R (1964) Bootlegged ecstasy. *JAMA* 187, 192.

Grinspoon, L, Bakalar, JB (1979) *Psychedelic Drugs Reconsidered*. Basic Books, New York.

Grinspoon, L, Bakalar, JB (1986) Can drugs be used to enhance the psychotherapeutic process? *Amer J Psychotherapy* 40, 393–404.

Grob, C, De Rios, MD (1992) Adolescent drug use in cross-cultural perspective. *J Drug Issues* 22, 121–138.

Grof, S (1980) *LSD Psychotherapy*. Hunter House, Pomona, CA.

Grof, S (1987) Spirituality, addiction, and western science: *ReVision* 10(2), 5–18.

Guerra, F (1967) Mexican phantastica—A study of the early ethnobotanical sources on hallucinogenic drugs. *Br J Addict* 61, 171–187.

Guerra, F (1971) *The Pre-Columbian Mind*. Seminar Press, London.

Guttman, E, Maclsy, WS (1936) Mescaline and depersonalization: Therapeutic experiments. *J Neurol Psychopath* 16, 193–212.

Harner, MJ (1973) The role of hallucinogenic plants in European witchcraft. In Harner MJ (Ed): *Hallucinogens and Shamanism*. pp. 125–150. London, Oxford University Press.

Heffter, A. (1897) Über Pellote. *Arch. Exp. Path. Pharmakol* 40, 418–425.

Hofmann, A (1985) LSD—*My Problem Child: Reflections on Sacred Drugs, Mysticism,* and Science. J. P. Tarcher, Los Angeles.

Hollister, LE, Shelton, J, Krieger, G (1969) A controlled comparison of lysergic diethylamide (LSD) and dextroamphetamine in alcoholics. *Amer J Psychiatry* 125, 1352–1357.

Huxley, A (1977) *Moksha: Writings on Psychedelics and the Visionary Experience*. J. P. Tarcher, Los Angeles.

Jacobs, BL (1984) *Hallucinogens: Neurochemical, Behavioral and Clinical Perspectives*. Raven Press, New York.

Jilek, WG (1971) From crazy witchdoctor to auxiliary psychotherapist: The changing image of the medicine man. *Psychiatrica Clinica* 4, 200–220.

Kluver, H (1928) *Mescal: The 'Divine' Plant and its Psychological Effects*. Kegan Paul, London.

LaBarre, W (1947) Primitive psychotherapy in Native American cultures: Peyotism and confession. *J Abnormal Soc Psychol* 42, 294–309.

Leary, T, Alpert, R (1962) The politics of consciousness. *Harvard Review* 1(4), 33–37.

Lee, MA, Shlain, B (1985) *Acid Dreams: The CIA, LSD and the Sixties Rebellion.* New York, Grove Weidenfeld.

Levine, J, Ludwig, AM (1967) The hypnodelic treatment technique. In HA Abramson (ed.), *The Use of LSD in Psychotherapy and Alcoholism.* New York, Bobbs-Merrill.

Ludwig, AM, Levine, J, Stark, LH (1970) *LSD and Alcoholism: A Clinical Study of Treatment Efficacy.* Springfield, Illinois, Charles C. Thomas.

Maclean, JR, Macdonald, DC, Byrne, UP, Hubbard. AM (1961) LSD in treatment of alcoholism and other psychiatric problems. *Quarterly J Studies Alcohol* 22, 34–45.

Marks, J (1979) *The Search for the "Manchurian Candidate."* New York, Dell.

Michelet, J (1965) *Satanism and Witchcraft: A Study in Medieval Superstition* (1862). Translated by A. R. Allinson. New York, Citadel.

Mitchell, SW (1896) Remarks on the effects of *Abhelonium lewinii* (the mescal button). *Br Med J* 2, 1625–1629.

Neill, JR (1987) "More than medical significance": LSD and American psychiatry 1953–1966. *J Psychoactive Drugs,* 19, 39–45.

Noll, R (1983) Shamanism and schizophrenia: A state-specific approach to the "schizophrenia metaphor" of shamanic states. *American Ethnologist* 10, 443–459.

O'Neil, M (1987) Magical healing, love magic and the Inquisition in late sixteenth-century Modena. In S. Haliczer (Ed): *Inquisition and Society in Early Modern Europe,* pp. 88–114. Croom Helm, London.

Osmond, H (1957) A review of the clinical effects of psychotomimetic agents. *Ann NY Acad Sci* 66, 418–434.

Rinkel, M, Denber, HCB (Eds) (1958) *Chemical Concepts of Psychosis.* Mc-Dowell, New York.

Schultes, RE (1938) The appeal of peyote (*Lophophora williaimsii*) as a medicine. *American Anthropologist* 40, 698–715.

Smart, RG, Storm, T, Baker EFW, Solursh, L (1966) A controlled study of lysergide in the treatment of alcoholism. *Quarterly J Studies Alcohol* 27, 469–482.

Stevens, J: Storming Heaven (1988) *LSD and the American Dream.* Harper and Row, New York.

Stockings, GT (1940) A clinical study of the mescaline psychosis, with special reference to the mechanism of the genesis of schizophrenia and other psychotic states. *J Mental Science* 86, 29–47.

Stoll, WA (1947) Lysergaure-diathylamid, ein Phantastikum aus der Mutterkorngruppe. *Schweizer Archiv fur Neurologie und Psychiatrie* 60, 279–323.

Strassman, RJ (1984) Adverse reactions to psychedelic drugs: A review of the literature. *J Nervous Mental Disease* 172, 577–595.

Strassman, RJ (1991) Human hallucinogenic drug research in the United States: A present-day case history and review of the process. *J Psychoactive Drugs* 23, 29–37.

Van Dusen, W, Wilson, W, Miners, W, Hook, H (1967) Treatment of alcoholism with lysergide. *Quarterly J Studies Alcohol* 28, 295–304.

Wasson, RG (1968) *Soma: Divine Mushroom of Immortality.* Harcourt, Brace and World, New York.

Wasson, RG, Ruck, CAP, Hofmann, A (1978) *The Road to Eleusis.* Harcourt, Brace, Jovanovich, New York.

Recommended Books

Collin, M: Altered State: *The Story of Ecstasy Culture and Acid House.* Serpent's Tail, London, 1997—*a chronicle of the rise of the rave culture and the dance drug movement in the United Kingdom.*

Dobkin-De Rios, M: *Hallucinogens: Cross-Cultural Perspectives.* University of New Mexico Press, Albuquerque, 1984—*an anthropologic survey of the use of mind-altering plants by indigenous societies around the world.*

Forte, R (ed.): *Entheogens and the Future of Religion.* Council on Spiritual Practices, San Francisco, 1997—*a collection of essays on the relation of hallucinogens to the religious experience.*

Grinspoon, L. and Bakalar, J.B: *Psychedelic Drugs Reconsidered.* Basic Books, New York, 1979—*an authoritative review of the history of hallucinogens, with particular emphasis on the examination of the record of hallucinogen research during the 1950s and 1960s.*

Grof, S and Halifax, J: *The Human Encounter with Death.* E. P. Dutton, New York, 1977—*a moving account of the authors' treatment of the psychological distress of dying cancer patients utilizing the synthetic hallucinogens, LSD and DPT.*

Grof, S: *LSD Psychotherapy.* Hunter House, Pomona, CA, 1980—*a comprehensive review of the theoretical framework and clinical experiences of the most accomplished hallucinogen researcher of his era.*

Harner, M: *Hallucinogens and Shamanism.* Oxford University Press, London, 1973—*a collection of anthropological essays on the shamanic structures employed by indigenous peoples when utilizing plant hallucinogens.*

Hofmann, A: *LSD: My Problem Child.* J. P. Tarcher, Los Angeles, 1983—*the autobiography of the famed Swiss research chemist and discoverer of the prototype twentieth-century hallucinogen.*

Huxley, A: *Moksha: Writings on Psychedelics and the Visionary Experience.* J. P. Tarcher, Los Angeles, 1977—*a collection of letters, essays and articles of the great English writer focusing on his fascination with hallucinogens during the final decade of his life.*

Ka-Tzetnik 135633: *Shivitti: A Vision.* Harper & Row, New York, 1989—*the compelling story of a concentration camp survivor reliving and healing his traumatic experiences while undergoing experimental LSD psychotherapy.*

Lee, M. A. and Shlain, B: *Acid Dreams: The CIA, LSD and the Sixties Rebellion.* Grove Weidenfeld, New York, 1985—*the fascinating story of the role of the U.S. government influencing research and cultural developments during the 1950s and 1960s.*

Luna, L. E. and Amaringo, P: *Ayahuasca Visions: The Religious Iconography of a Peruvian Shaman.* North Atlantic Books, Berkeley, CA, 1991—*a collaborative effort between an anthropologist and mestizo ayahuasca healer in the Amazon, with numerous color prints depicting the mythologies surrounding the use of ayahuasca in South America.*

McKenna, T: *True Hallucinations.* Harper Collins, San Francisco, 1993—*the intriguing tale of two brothers in search of the mythical shamanic hallucinogen of the Amazon.*

Metzner, R: *Ayahuasca: Hallucinogens, Consciousness and the Spirit of Nature.* Thunder's Mouth Press, New York, 1999—*an examination of the biochemical, ethnobotanical and psychological dimensions of the ayahuasca experience, along with numerous firsthand accounts.*

Narby, J: *The Cosmic Serpent: DNA and the Origins of Knowledge.* Jeremy P. Tarcher/Putnam, New York, 1998—*the fascinating account of the experiences of a Swiss anthropologist in Peru, and the startling connection he makes between ayahuasca-induced consciousness and the field of molecular biology.*

Ott, J: *Pharmacotheon: Entheogenic Drugs, Their Plant Sources and History.* Natural Products, Kenniwick, WA, 1993—*the densely detailed compilation of the history, ethnobotany and biochemistry of a variety of plant and synthetic hallucinogens.*

Shultes, R. E. and Hofmann, A: *Plants of the Gods: Their Sacred, Healing and Hallucinogenic Powers.* Healing Arts Press, Rochester, VT, 1992—*the authoritative review of the ethnobotany, chemistry, history and mythology of plant hallucinogens, prepared by two eminent investigators.*

Stafford, P: *Psychedelics Encyclopedia.* Ronin Publishing, Berekely, CA, 1992—*a comprehensive source book on the psychological, biological, and cultural aspects of hallucingens.*

Stevens, J: *Storming Heaven: LSD and the American Dream.* Harper & Row, New York, 1988—*the compelling cultural history of the role played by hallucinogens during the 1950s and 1960s.*

Sources and Permissions

Chapter 1 is from "A Conversation with Albert Hofmann," in the *MAPS Bulletin* 8(3):30–33, 1998. Reprinted with permission from the Multidisciplinary Association for Psychedelic Studies (MAPS), 2105 Robinson Avenue, Sarasota, Florida 34232.

Chapter 2 is from "Molecular Mysticism: The Role of Psychoactive Substances in Transformations of Consciousness," in *Shaman's Drum* 12(2):15–21, 1988. Reprinted with permission from the author.

Chapter 3 is from "Psychedelic Society," in *Entheogens and the Future of Religion,* Council on Spiritual Practices, San Francisco, 1997. Reprinted with permission from the Council on Spiritual Practices.

Chapter 4 is from "Two Classic Trips: Jean-Paul Sartre and Adelle Davis," in *Gnosis Magazine* 26(1):34–41, 1993. Reprinted with permission from the author.

Chapter 5 is from "The Good Friday Experiment," in *Cleansing the Doors of Perception,* Jeremy P. Tarcher/Putnam, New York, 2000. Reprinted with permission from the author.

Chapter 6 is from "Mysticism: Contemplative and Chemical," in *Gnosis Magazine* 26(1):19–21, 1993. Reprinted with permission from the author.

Chapter 7 is from "Drugs and Jewish Spirituality: That was Then, This is Now," in *Tikkun* 14(3):39–43, 1999. Reprinted from Tikkun.

Chapter 8 is from "Using Psychedelics Wisely," in *Gnosis Magazine* 26(1)26–30, 1993. Reprinted with permission from the author.

Chapter 9 is from "Successful Outcome of a single LSD Treatment in a Chronically Dysfunctional Man," in the *MAPS Bulletin* 9(2):11–14, 1999. Reprinted with permission from the Multidisciplinary Association for Psychedelic Studies (MAPS), 2105 Robinson Ave, Sarasota, Florida 34232.

Chapter 10 is from "Sitting for Sessions: Dharma & DMT Research," in *Tricycle: The Buddhist Review* 6(1):81–87, 1996. Reprinted with permission from the author.

Chapter 11 is from "The Psychedelic Vision at the Turn of the Millennium: Discussion with Andrew Weil, M.D.," in the *MAPS Bulletin* 8(1):28–37, 1998. Reprinted with permission from the Multidisciplinary Association for Psychedelic Studies (MAPS), 2105 Robinson Ave, Sarasota, Florida 34232.

Chapter 12 is from "Making Friends with Cancer and Ayahuasca," in *Shaman's Drum* 55(2):32–39, 2000. Reprinted with permission from the author.

Chapter 13 is from "Psychoactive Plants and Ethnopsychiatric Medicines of the Matsigenka," in the *Journal of Psychoactive Drugs* 30(4):321–332, 1998. Reprinted with permission from the *Journal of Psychoactive Drugs*.

Chapter 14 is from "Shamans and Scientists," in *Intrinsic Value and Integrity of Plants in the Context of Genetic Engineering,* 9–11 May 2000, Doruach, Switzerland.

Chapter 15 is from "Ritual Approaches to Working with Sacred Medicine Plants: An Interview with Ralph Metzner, Ph.D.," in *Shaman's Drum* 51(2):19–29, 1999. Reprinted with permission from the author.

Appendix A is from "The Psychology of Ayahuasca," in *Ayahuasca: Hallucinogens, Consciousness and the Spirit of Nature,* Thunder's Mouth Press, New York, 1999. Reprinted with permission from the author.

Appendix B is from "Deconstructing Ecstasy: The Politics of MDMA Research," in *Addiction Research,* 2000.

Appendix C is from "Psychiatric Research with Hallucinogens: What Have We Learned?" in the *Heffter Review of Psychedelic Research* 1:8–19, 1998. Reprinted with permission of the Heffter Research Institute.

Contributors

Lawrence Bush is the author of *American Torah Toons: 54 Illustrated Commentaries* and co-editor of *Jews, a new magazine of visual art and literature.*

Gary Fisher, Ph.D., is a retired UCLA psychologist who collaborated on approved clinical research with hallucinogens in the 1960s. These studies examined the effectiveness of hallucinogens in the treatment of schizophrenia, autism and the psychological distress of terminal medical illness.

Albert Hofmann, Ph.D., is the retired director of the Pharmaceutical-Chemical Research Laboratories of Sandoz, Ltd., in Basel, Switzerland. He is the discoverer of lysergic acid diethylamide (LSD) and the first to synthesize psilocybin, the active constituent of the Mexican sacred mushroom. He is the author of numerous chemical and pharmaceutical research books. With Dr. Richard Evans Schultes of Harvard University, he is the co-author of *Plants of the Gods* and *The Botany and Chemistry of Hallucinogens,* and he is the co-author with R. G. Wasson and Carl Ruck of *The Road to Eleusis.* Dr. Hoffman has also authored an autobiography, entitled *LSD: My Problem Child.*

Terence McKenna was a scholar of the ethnobotany of the Amazon Basin and shamanism, who died in April, 2000. Together with his brother Dennis McKenna, he authored *The Invisible Landscape* and *Psilocybin: The Magic Mushroom Grower's Guide.* Additional books written by Terence McKenna include *The Archaic Revival* and *True Hallucinations.*

Ralph Metzner, Ph.D., is a professor of psychology at the California Institute of Integral Studies in San Francisco. He is the co-author of *The Psychedelic Experience,* and the author of *Know Your Type, Opening to Inner Light, The Well of Remembrance, The Unfolding Self* and *Green Psychology.* He is also the editor of *Ayahuasca: Hallucinogens, Consciousness and the Spirit of Nature.*

Jeremy Narby, Ph.D., is an anthropologist who has done extensive field work in the Peruvian Amazon. He is the author of *The Cosmic Serpent: DNA and the Origins of Knowledge.*

Thomas Riedlinger is a fellow of the Linnean Society of London and former associate in ethnomycology at the Harvard Botanical Museum. He is the editor of *The Sacred Mushroom Seeker: Essays for R. Gordon Wasson.*

Glenn Shepard, Ph.D., is an anthropologist who has conducted ethnobotanical research among indigenous tribes of the Peruvian Amazon, documented in the Discovery Channel films, *Spirits of the Rainforest* and *The Spirit Hunters.*

Huston Smith, Ph.D., is a professor emeritus of comparative religion at the University of California, Berkeley. In 1996, Bill Moyers devoted a five-part PBS special, *The Wisdom of Faith with Huston Smith,* to his life and work. He is the author of *Cleansing the Doors of Perception: The Religious Significance of Entheogenic Plants and Chemicals.*

Myron Stolaroff is a veteran researcher in the field of hallucinogens. Between 1960 and 1970 he was the director of the *International Foundation for Advanced Study,* a research group conducting approved clinical studies with LSD and mescaline. He is the author of *Thanatos to Eros* and *The Secret Chief.*

Rick Strassman, M.D., is a former associate professor of psychiatry at the University of New Mexico, where he developed FDA-approved clinical research studies with DMT and psilocybin. He is the author of *DMT: The Spirit Molecule.*

Donald Topping, Ph.D., is a professor emeritus in Linguistics at the University of Hawaii, and President of the Drug Policy Forum of Hawaii.

Roger Walsh, M.D., Ph.D., is a professor of psychiatry, philosophy and anthropology at the University of California, Irvine. He is the author of *The Spirit of Shamanism, Staying Alive: The Psychology of Human Survival* and *Essential Spirituality: The 7 Central Practices to Awakening Heart and Mind.* He is the co-editor with Frances Vaughan of *Paths Beyond Ego: The Transpersonal Vision.*

Andrew Weil, M.D., is a professor of internal medicine at the University of Arizona. He is the founder of the Program for Integrative Medicine, which trains physicians in alternative medicine. He is the author of *Spontaneous Healing, Eight Weeks to Optimum Health, The Marriage of the Sun and the Moon* and *The Natural Mind.*

About the Editor

Charles S. Grob, M.D., is Director of the Division of Child and Adolescent Psychiatry at Harbor-UCLA Medical Center, and Professor of Psychiatry and Pediatrics at the UCLA School of Medicine. He did his undergraduate work at Oberlin College and Columbia University, and obtained a B.S. from Columbia in 1975. He received his M.D. from the State University of New York, Downstate Medical Center, in 1979. Prior to his appointment at UCLA, Dr. Grob has held teaching and clinical positions at the University of California at Irvine, College of Medicine and The Johns Hopkins University School of Medicine, Departments of Psychiatry and Pediatrics. He conducted the first government-approved psychobiological research study of MDMA, and was the principal investigator of an international biomedical-psychiatric research project in the Brazilian Amazon of the plant hallucinogen, ayahuasca. He has published numerous articles in medical and psychiatric journals and collected volumes. He is a founding board member of the Heffter Research Institute.

A NEW
CONSCIOUSNESS
READER

This New Consciousness Reader is part of a series of original and classic writing by renowned experts on leading-edge concepts in personal development, psychology, spiritual growth, and healing. Other books in this series include:

Sacred Sorrows: Embracing and Transforming Depression
EDITED BY JOHN E. NELSON, M.D., AND ANDREA NELSON, PSY.D.

The Spirit of Writing: Classic and Contemporary Essays
Celebrating the Writing Life
EDITED BY MARK ROBERT WALDMAN

Spiritual Emergency: When Personal Transformation Becomes a Crisis
EDITED BY STANISLAV GROF, M.D., AND CHRISTINA GROF

The Truth about the Truth: De-Confusing the Postmodern World
EDITED BY WALTER TRUETT ANDERSON

What Survives? Contemporary Exploration of Life after Death
EDITED BY GARY DOORE, PH.D.